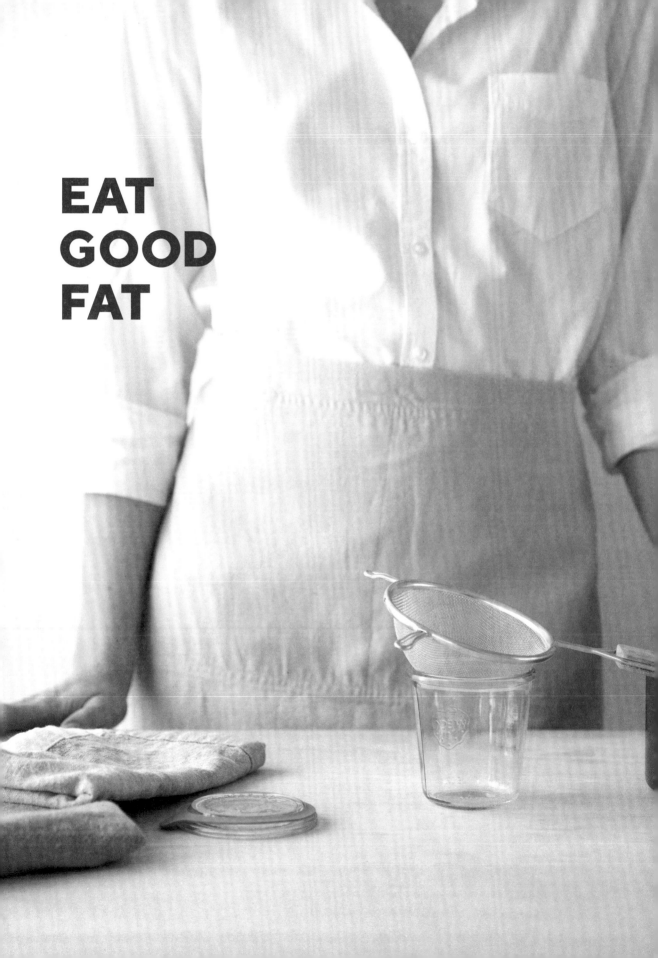

EAT
GOOD
FAT

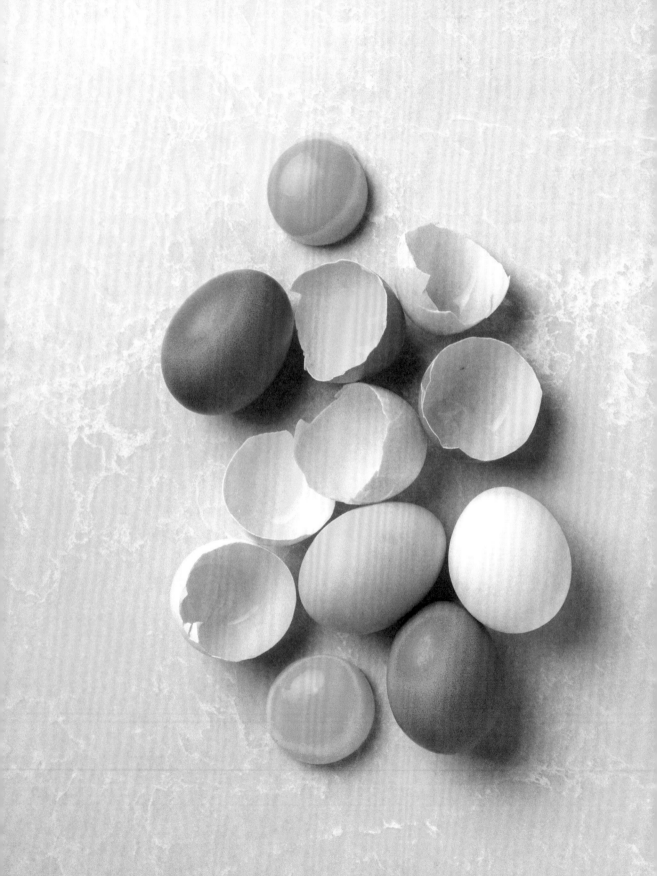

EAT GOOD FAT

Nourish Your Body with Over 100 Healthy, Fat-Fuelled Recipes

Lee Capatina

PENGUIN
an imprint of Penguin Canada, a division of
Penguin Random House Canada Limited

Canada • USA • UK • Ireland • Australia • New Zealand • India •
South Africa • China

First published 2020

www.penguinrandomhouse.ca

Library and Archives Canada Cataloguing in Publication

Title: Eat good fat : nourish your body with over 100 healthy,
fat-fuelled recipes / Capatina Lee.
Names: Lee, Capatina, author.
Identifiers: Canadiana (print) 20200173820 | Canadiana (ebook)
20200173863 | ISBN 9780735237971 (hardcover) |
ISBN 9780735237988 (HTML)
Subjects: LCSH: Ketogenic diet. | LCSH: Oils and fats, Edible. |
LCSH: Lipids in human nutrition. | LCGFT: Cookbooks.
Classification: LCC TX714 .L44 2021 | DDC 641.5/638—dc23

Cover and interior design by Lisa Jager
Cover and interior photography by Lauren Miller
Food styling by Dara Sutin
Prop styling by Rayna Marlee Schwartz

10 9 8 7 6 5 4 3 2 1

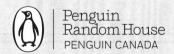

Penguin
Random House
PENGUIN CANADA

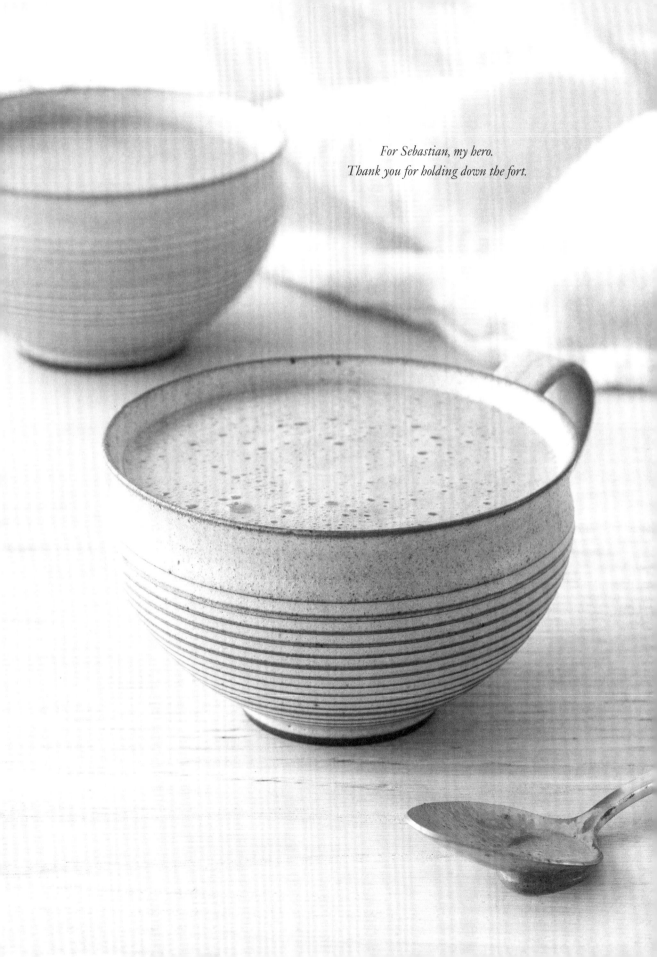

For Sebastian, my hero.
Thank you for holding down the fort.

✦ Contents

Morning Eats

Soups and Salads

Mains and Sides

Snacks and Small Bites

Drinks

Desserts

Staples

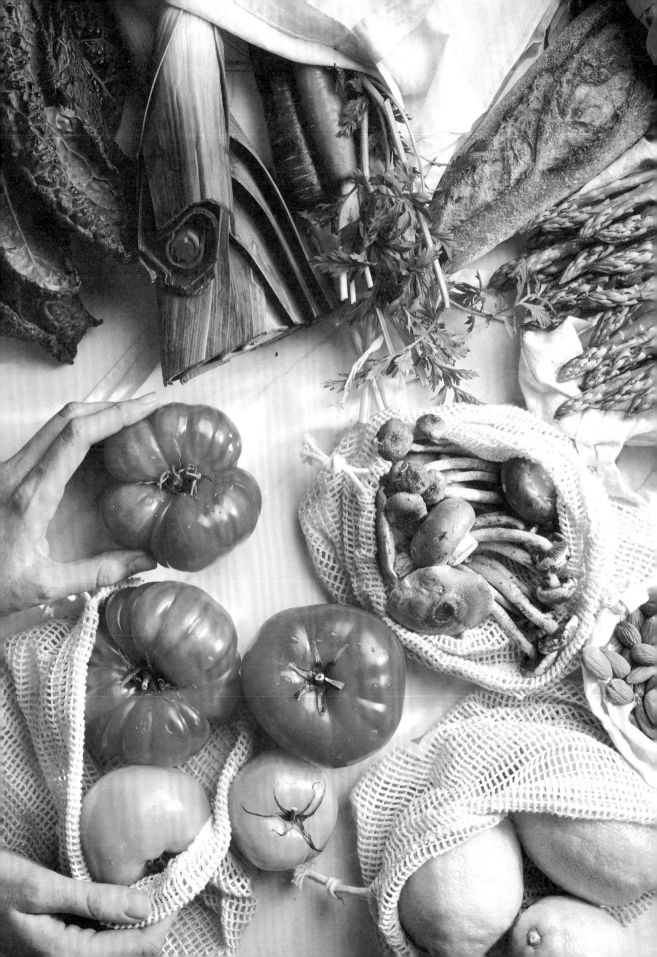

Introduction

When I was thirteen years old, I was scouted to become a model. Shortly after, I signed with a Toronto-based agency that was known for launching "new faces." What followed were years of jet-setting to places like Tokyo, Singapore, Milan, Paris, Auckland, and New York—all before I turned eighteen. Modelling helped me gain confidence and become more independent, and it shaped who I am today, but it came at a cost.

I was taught that my self-worth was tied to how I looked, regardless of how I felt. Throughout my career, I was under constant pressure to lose weight by whatever means possible. The idea was to follow a low-fat diet and intense workout regimen with the hopes of fitting into standard-size sample garments for shows. This consisted of eating foods that made me feel hungry and deprived. In extreme cases, when I had to lose extra weight quickly (such as before fashion week), I would restrict myself further by going on detoxes like the Master Cleanse or Cabbage Soup Diet. These fad diets caused me to have headaches, low energy, and uncontrollable food cravings. This led to cycles of binge eating and subsequent weight gain—putting me right back where I started. While low-fat diets may have short-term benefits, they don't work over the long term. After several years of yo-yo dieting and feeling terrible, I decided to quit modelling once and for all.

I began soul searching for a happier, healthier way of life. I moved to Brooklyn, New York, where I was introduced to a thriving local food community. I started shopping at farmers markets, became friends with entrepreneurs who had small food businesses, and learned about new things like urban farming and beekeeping. This planted the seed for what would become an enduring passion for healthy food and sustainability. One day, a friend brought me to a seminar on Ayurveda, traditional Indian medicine. This is where I first learned about ghee

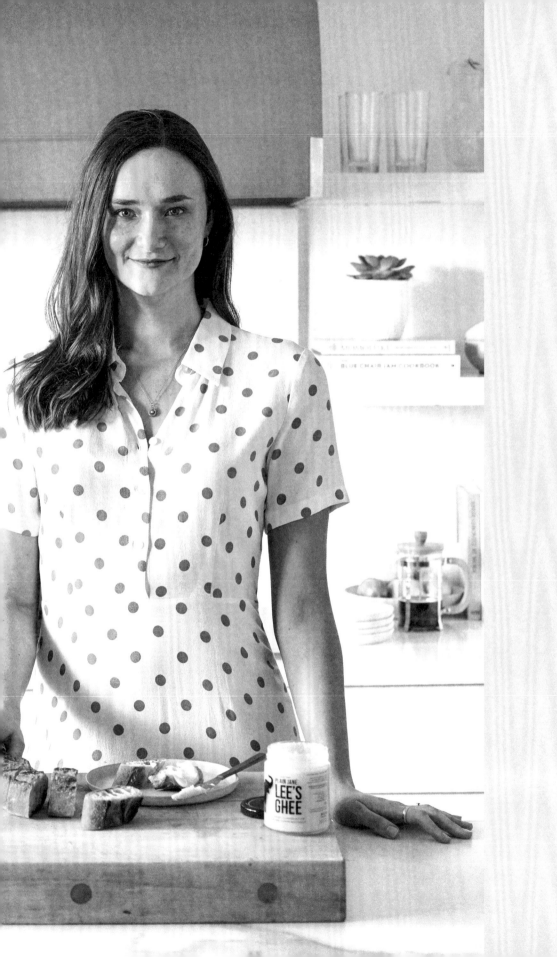

and its benefits. I was fascinated and taught myself to make it at home shortly after. I started using it in my everyday cooking: for frying eggs, adding to smoothies, and smearing on toast. I fell in love with its buttery flavour and the nourishment it provided. This was the beginning of a new way of thinking about fats and a lifelong affair with ghee.

Eager to learn more about Ayurveda and sustainability, I travelled to India to work on an organic farm. There, I found myself surrounded by people from around the world who were just as keen as I was to connect with food in a meaningful way. I loved working the land and felt a sense of total freedom in the fields, but the place I found myself drawn to the most was the farm kitchen. I learned how to cook simple Ayurvedic recipes, such as kitchari, with fresh ingredients like turmeric, ginger, ghee, and vegetables grown on the farm. After several weeks on the farm and travelling throughout India, I became homesick and felt the desire to go home to Canada and plant my roots.

I enrolled in nutrition school in Toronto to become a certified holistic nutritionist, but the universe had other plans for me. The summer before school began, I was showing a friend how to make ghee, and he jokingly suggested that I start a company called Lee's Ghee. I took his suggestion to heart and began selling mason jars full of organic ghee at a local farmers market. I didn't really consider that this summer gig might have the potential to turn into a full-fledged business. When school began, the teachers and students found out about my ghee and wanted to get their hands on it. At the same time, I was getting phone calls from retailers who had heard about what I was doing and wanted to stock it on their shelves. I felt a powerful pull to follow this path, so I put school on hold and scrambled to find a commercial kitchen to fill all the orders that I was receiving. I had no business degree, no money, and frankly no idea what I was doing, but I felt that I had finally found my calling. I decided then and there that I would do whatever it took to pursue my passion.

Since then, the business has grown in ways I never could have imagined. The company evolved from being called Lee's Ghee to Lee's Provisions to encompass other product lines, such as our line of Good Fat Blends made of coconut oil and ghee and our organic tulsi wellness teas—with many more products launching in the future! I've worked tirelessly to create a business that nourishes people with good fats, supports farmers using sustainable agricultural practices, and gives back to causes I believe in. I have convinced hundreds of stores to carry my products, sold thousands of jars of ghee across the country, and educated many about the benefits of eating good fat. But I am not slowing down now—the next step is to convince the entire world to eat good fat!

As a holistic nutritionist, I have been obsessed with learning about health and nutrition since my early twenties and continue to take courses whenever I have time. My passion is for healthy fats and eating whole foods. The Food and Drug Administration and the Canadian Food Inspection Agency have not evaluated the information in this book and the book is not intended to diagnose, treat, or cure any disease. You should always consult with your doctor before making drastic changes to your diet.

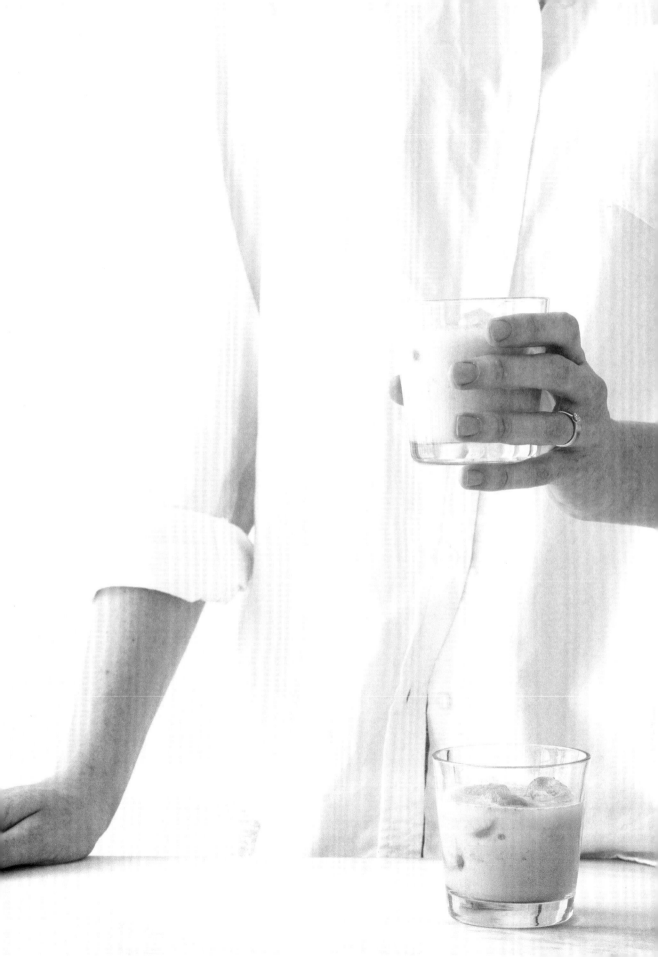

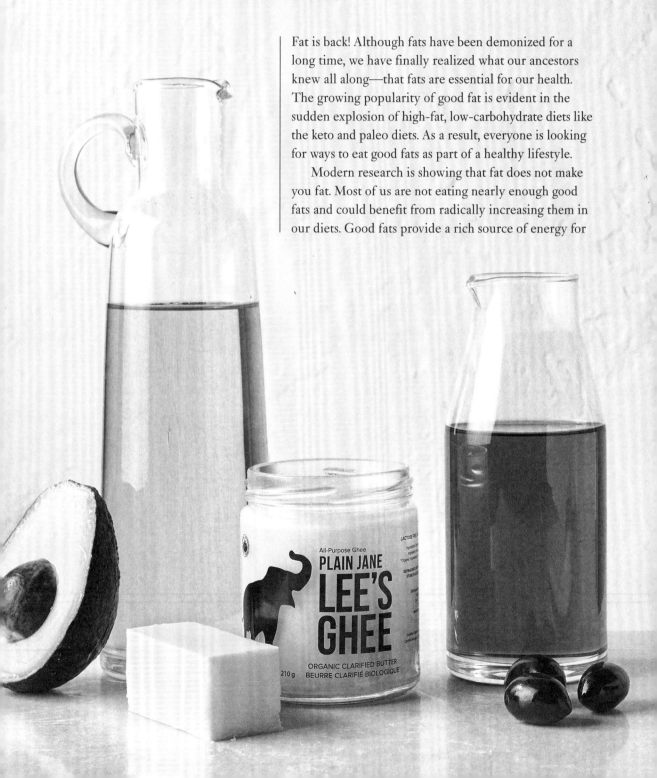

About the Book—
Fat Is Back!

Fat is back! Although fats have been demonized for a long time, we have finally realized what our ancestors knew all along—that fats are essential for our health. The growing popularity of good fat is evident in the sudden explosion of high-fat, low-carbohydrate diets like the keto and paleo diets. As a result, everyone is looking for ways to eat good fats as part of a healthy lifestyle.

Modern research is showing that fat does not make you fat. Most of us are not eating nearly enough good fats and could benefit from radically increasing them in our diets. Good fats provide a rich source of energy for the mind and body, balance blood sugar levels, help with the absorption of vitamins, lower bad cholesterol, and keep you full for longer. Most importantly, fats make food taste great!

Eat Good Fat makes eating healthy simple with 100 delicious recipes that use whole food ingredients and plenty of good fats. Each recipe is part of a road map that will guide you in using fats correctly and in a healthy way. To accomplish this, I've been mindful of carefully considering both the cooking properties and the flavours of each type of fat. Whereas you can get the most goodness from certain fats, such as olive oil, in their unheated form, others really shine when cooking at high temperatures. For example, coconut oil and ghee can both be used at high temperatures, but frying eggs in coconut oil may not produce the best flavour. Cooking eggs in ghee, on the other hand, adds an irresistible butteriness and is a total game changer.

I hope that by making the recipes in this book, you will gain confidence in using good fats in your kitchen to cook healthy, delicious meals at home that you can feel good about. Eating healthy food does not have to be complicated or overwhelming. It begins with the small decisions we make every single day—it begins with eating good fat!

My philosophy is that it is not the diet you follow but the quality of what you eat that counts. My body thrives on eating a variety of whole foods, including complex carbohydrates, in addition to healthy protein, an abundance of vegetables, and good fats. My husband, Sebastian, on the other hand, eats a mostly paleo diet that includes plenty of good fats, high-quality animal protein, and a lot of vegetables while limiting most carbohydrates in the form

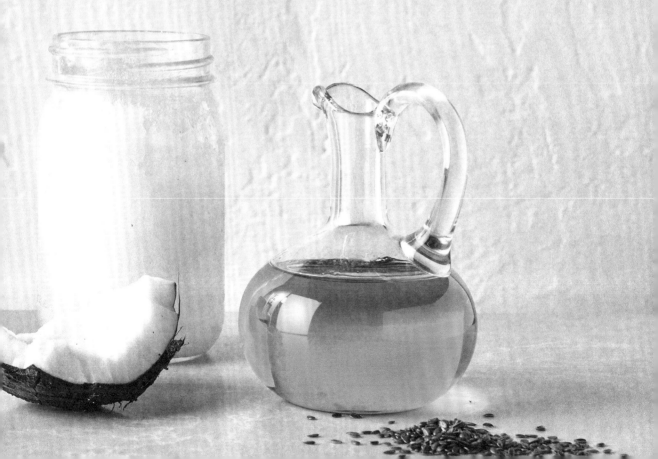

of bread, legumes, and grains. It would be complicated to make separate meals, so I like to cook in a way that is easily adapted. It can be as simple as leaving out the English muffin when having Eggs Florentine with Smoked Salmon and Ghee Hollandaise (page 64) for breakfast. The important thing is to know your own body and what makes you feel best. Each of us is unique, and we all have different needs.

The recipes in this book were designed to have a broad appeal to anyone looking to embrace good fat (in all its delicious glory). I've made a point to include variations wherever appropriate and encourage you to adjust the recipes to suit your individual lifestyle choices or dietary restrictions. My general rule is that if you are using whole food ingredients and cooking from scratch, you are off to a good start!

You can find many of the ingredients for the recipes in this book along the perimeter or in the natural aisle of a well-stocked grocery store; the rest of the ingredients can be found on a trip to the farmers market or health food store. If available to you, I highly recommend sourcing eggs, dairy products, and meat directly from producers who can attest that their animals live in a natural environment and can roam outdoors. Although higher welfare animal products come with a higher price tag, the truth is that you really get what you pay for. Meat, poultry, eggs, and dairy from pasture-raised or organic animals not only taste much better, but also provide far superior nutritional profiles when compared to their factory-farmed counterparts.

This book is intended to make it easy for you to incorporate good fats into your daily cooking. Each chapter includes delicious, nutrient-dense recipes that are simple to make and will help keep you feeling satiated and energized all day long!

Morning Eats

This chapter consists of recipes that will get your day started off on the right foot. In the morning, it is especially important to eat a balanced breakfast that incorporates healthy protein, good fats, and complex carbohydrates. This combination is essential to stabilize your energy levels and keep you satisfied until lunchtime. Recipes like Crispy Sweet Potato Egg Nests (page 60) and Buckwheat Chia Pudding with Almond Butter Drizzle (page 55) deliver all that and more! There are both sweet and savoury breakfast options—many, like Ghee Toast (page 38), are quick and easy enough to make during the week, whereas others, like Eggs Florentine with Smoked Salmon and Ghee Hollandaise (page 64), are best reserved for leisurely weekend brunches.

Soups
and Salads

Unlike many soups and salads, these ones will not leave you feeling hungry afterwards. They contain plenty of good fats and healthy protein. I use coconut milk and ghee to make soups like Lobster and Wild Salmon Bisque (page 91) unctuous, velvety, and creamy. Homemade Bone Broth (page 272) is the perfect base for a soup and adds staying power and collagen—an essential nutrient for your skin and gut health. The salads, such as Avocado Rocket Salad with Mustard Lemon Vinaigrette (page 101), are full of nourishing ingredients like sheep's milk cheese, avocado, nuts, and seeds. Some of the salads hold their own as a main course, whereas others are better suited for serving alongside any grilled protein at lunch or dinner. I often like to pair a soup and salad for a light, energizing lunch.

Mains
and Sides

This chapter is a collection of main courses and side dishes that are hearty and nutrient dense. All of these recipes include a balance of healthy protein, good fats, and complex carbohydrates. I made a point to include plenty of main courses in this book, as they form the bulk of what we eat every day. Some of them can be made on a single sheet pan, like Sheet Pan Sausage Dinner with Caramelized Cabbage and Red Onion (page 140), or in one pot, like One-Pot Sweet Potato, Spinach, and Chickpea Stew (page 167). Others are more involved and require performing steps ahead of time. The sides are simple additions that help round out a meal by adding extra vegetables, fibre, and nutrients. In addition to recipes that incorporate a variety of healthy animal proteins, there are a few vegetarian options in this chapter, like Millet Risotto with Crispy Roasted Mushrooms and a Poached Egg (page 116).

Snacks and
Small Bites

This chapter features small bites that are perfect for taking with you to work, enjoying as an afternoon snack, or serving as an appetizer. I like to make a batch of Tahini-Coconut Fat Balls (page 187) to snack on for a clean energy boost mid-afternoon, and I serve savoury spreads like Kalamata Olive Tapenade (page 200) with nutrient-dense Seedy Almond Pulp Crackers (page 192) as a fat-fuelled appetizer. I've also been known to eat appetizers as snacks and to serve snacks as appetizers. The truth is, there are no rules, and you are free to enjoy the recipes in any way you want!

Drinks

This chapter includes fat-fuelled smoothies, lattes, and drinks that are focused on providing energy to your mind and body. They can be made first thing in the morning, before a workout, or during an afternoon hanger slump—whenever you want something light and energizing to tide you over until your next meal. Although I focus on using good fats as the primary source of energy in all of these drinks, I like to amp up my Almond Butter Date Shake (page 217) and I Love You So Matcha (page 227) by adding adaptogenic herbs such as energy-boosting maca or stress-busting ashwagandha. I also highly recommend adding a scoop of collagen protein for its renowned skin and gut-loving benefits.

Desserts

Although sweets are best consumed in moderation, we all need to treat ourselves some-times. This chapter includes some of my favourite desserts. I like to serve the Cardamom Date Cake with Goat Cheese Frosting (page 255) with tea or coffee during an afternoon break. We always make Sebastian's German Cherry Cake (page 252) for special occasions, and I love eating leftover Coconut Black Rice Pudding (page 263) for breakfast! The desserts derive their natural sweetness from ingredients like Medjool dates, maple syrup, and honey. Since the sweeteners used are unprocessed and unrefined, they contain the nutrients required to metabolize the sugars, while the good fats and fibre in the recipes work to keep blood sugar in check. This means you can feel good about consuming these desserts on spe-cial occasions. Besides, you should never feel guilty for indulging a bit.

Staples

This chapter includes staple recipes to have on hand for adding healthy fats and flavour to the recipes in the book. Recipes include some of my favourite kitchen staples like Plain Jane Ghee (page 271), Fresh Pesto (page 276), and Homemade Almond Butter (page 275). I also outline three easy, straight-forward ways to cook your eggs to amp up the nutrition of any meal. These recipes form the basis of many recipes in the book, so you will want to refer back to this chapter often.

Dietary Restrictions

As you work your way through this book, you will notice that I have used some of the following dietary labels at the beginning of each recipe. This offers clarity on which recipes are suitable for those with dietary restrictions. I hope you will find them useful.

Dairy-Free These recipes are free of all dairy products, except for ghee (clarified butter). When ghee is made, the milk sugars and protein are removed from the butter, rendering it 99 percent lactose-free and casein-free. This makes it safe for those with lactose intolerance and dairy sensitivities. Unless a person is extremely sensitive or allergic to dairy, ghee will normally not cause problems. If you are extremely sensitive or allergic to dairy, I recommend checking with your doctor before consuming ghee. Alternatively, you can always use coconut oil as a substitute.

Gluten-Free These recipes are free of all gluten, making them safe for those with gluten sensitivity and celiac disease.

Grain-Free These recipes are free of all grains, including gluten-free grains and pseudograins.

Nut-Free These recipes are free of all nuts, making them safe for children to bring to school and for those with nut allergies.

Keto-Friendly These recipes are primarily free of carbohydrate-based foods such as grains, legumes, sugary fruit, root vegetables, rice, bread, alcohol, potatoes, and sweeteners. However, a small amount of carbohydrates (20 to 50 g per day) is allowed on the keto diet, so the recipes may include low-sugar fruit like plantains or berries.

Paleo-Friendly These recipes adhere to the paleo diet. They are free of grains, legumes, dairy products (excluding ghee), alcohol, and bread and include some carbohydrate-based foods such as root vegetables, fruit, and natural sweeteners like maple syrup, coconut sugar, and honey.

Vegan These recipes are free of all animal products, including meat, poultry, eggs, fish, dairy products, honey, cheese, and so on. All vegan recipes are vegetarian by default.

Vegetarian These recipes are free of meat, poultry, and fish, but they may contain vegetarian animal products like eggs, dairy products, honey, or cheese.

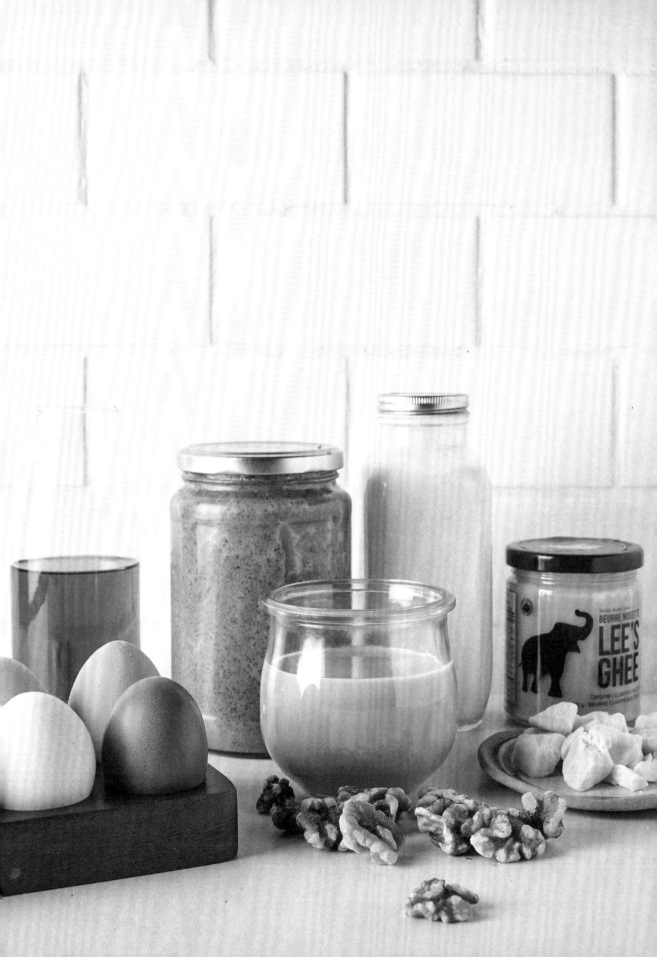

Fat:
The Good,
the Bad,
and the Ugly

The fat scare began in the 1970s when researchers discovered that cholesterol was a risk factor for heart disease and that saturated fats raise cholesterol. We were advised to avoid fat and replace our butter, full-fat dairy, red meat, and egg yolks with diet products like margarine, low-fat dairy, lean meats, and egg whites. In an attempt to avoid heart disease, low-fat diets became all the rage, and we began to replace dietary fats with refined carbohydrates and sugar. As a result of our changing diets, rates of obesity and diabetes began to rise steadily. Avoiding fats and replacing them with low-fat, sugar-filled substitutes was one of the biggest nutrition mistakes we've ever made.

The other problem was that we lumped all fats together, failing to recognize that there are both *bad* fats and *good* fats. Bad fats come from highly processed seed and vegetable oils, hydrogenation, and factory-farmed animal products. These fats are highly inflammatory and cause more harm than good. Good fats come from nuts and seeds, pasture-raised animal products, wild-caught fish, and fatty fruits like olives, avocados, and coconuts. These natural, unprocessed fats have stood the test of time and are full of inherent goodness and nutritional value. It can be confusing to know which fats fall into which category. Throughout this chapter, I will set the record straight and outline which fats you can eat without fear and which ones you should avoid.

Bad Fats

These are the sources of fat that you should avoid to the best of your abilities. They are highly processed and can cause inflammation in excess. If an oil has been refined or hydrogenated in any way, you don't want it in your kitchen.

- Chemically refined seed oils, such as cottonseed, grapeseed, sunflower, and safflower
- Chemically refined vegetable oils, such as canola, soybean, corn, and peanut
- Hydrogenated oils found in margarine, vegetable shortening, vegetable ghee, and some vegan products
- Factory-farmed meat, poultry, fish, eggs, and dairy products

Most vegetable and seed oils require extensive processing to extract. They are polyunsaturated fats that naturally have a higher amount of omega-6 fatty acids and are neutralized, filtered, or deodorized using harsh chemicals. These oils are very cheap to produce and are falsely promoted as being heart healthy and high in omega-3 fats. However, when they are extracted in this way, it destroys their omega-3 fats and oxidizes the oils, causing them to become inflammatory. Seed and vegetable oils are very delicate and should be used only as finishing oils if they are cold pressed, organic, and unrefined.

Hydrogenated oils are to be avoided at all costs, as they are further processed from refined vegetable oils. Hydrogenation forces hydrogen gas into oil at high pressure, making it solid and shelf stable. During this process, healthy fats are turned into a new type of fat, called artificial trans fat. Trans fats are incredibly inflammatory and are known to be a significant contributor to heart disease. They also raise bad cholesterol levels while lowering good cholesterol levels. Many processed foods contain hydrogenated oils and therefore contain trans fats.

I've included factory-farmed animal products as bad fats because the animal products that come out of factory farms have a completely different nutrition profile than organic, pasture-raised animal products or wild-caught fish. There is research to show that pasture-raised meats are not only significantly better for the environment, but also nutritionally superior to grain-fed, factory-farmed meats. Feeding animals grains yields meat with higher levels of omega-6 fatty acids and lower levels of omega-3 fatty acids. A healthy ratio of omega-6s to omega-3s is lower than 4:1, and you will find that ratio in grass-fed meat. In grain-fed meat and farmed fish, the ratio can be as high as 20:1. This is one reason why our modern diets are so much higher in omega-6s than omega-3s.

A Word on Cholesterol

Cholesterol is an essential component of cell membranes and is required by the body for many functions, such as the production of hormones. It is produced naturally by the liver and by digesting the food we eat. There is no such thing as good cholesterol and bad cholesterol, but cholesterol is carried by two different types of lipoproteins called low-density lipoprotein (LDL) and high-density lipoprotein (HDL), which can be good or bad.

The good kind of lipoprotein, HDL, does not easily stick to arteries and has been linked to a lower risk of heart disease. The bad kind of lipoprotein, LDL, may not be all bad after all, as there is a distinction between large and small LDL. Research has shown that small LDL particles can go through the artery wall and may be linked to heart disease. On the other hand, large LDL particles are mostly benign. Therefore, small LDL particles are the ones we should fear. These small LDL particles are increased by eating refined sugar, refined carbohydrates, and trans fats.

Healthy fats can help balance cholesterol levels. As most people know, polyunsaturated (omega-3 and omega-6) fats and monounsaturated fats lower total cholesterol levels, which is a good thing. Although saturated fat raises total cholesterol levels, it may not be as harmful as previously thought, because it transforms small LDL particles (harmful) to large LDL particles (benign) and slightly increases HDL.

The body has an inherent ability to balance its cholesterol levels for optimal health. However, this process can be hindered by poor diet or genetic disposition. To help the body naturally flush out excess cholesterol, it is essential to eat plenty of fibre in the form of whole grains, fresh vegetables, nuts, and fruit and to eliminate trans fats, refined carbohydrates, and refined sugar from your diet.

Good Fats

The good fats come from whole foods and their oils that are minimally processed. These are monounsaturated, polyunsaturated, and saturated fats that are found in nature and have not been damaged through processing, leaving their original nutrients and fat profiles intact. You can eat these foods knowing that the healthy fats they contain will support your overall health and well-being.

- Coconuts and virgin coconut oil
- Avocados and avocado oil
- Olives and extra-virgin olive oil

- Wild-caught, fatty fish
- Pasture-raised or organic eggs
- Organic or grass-fed meats and dairy
- Nuts and nut butter
- Seeds and seed butter
- Dark chocolate and cacao butter

Monounsaturated Fats (Omega-9)

Monounsaturated fats may protect against heart disease and raise the levels of good cholesterol while lowering the levels of bad cholesterol. The best sources of mono-unsaturated fats are avocados, olives, eggs, and certain nuts, but these fats are also found in butter and chicken fat in smaller amounts. An easy way to up your intake of monounsaturated fats is to regularly snack on macadamia nuts, almonds, pistachios, and cashews. These nuts are also loaded with protein and fibre, making them great to have on hand for any occasion. To sum it up, monounsaturated fats are all-around incredibly good for you, so go nuts (pun intended) and enjoy them every day!

Polyunsaturated Fats (Omega-3 and Omega-6)

There are two main types of polyunsaturated fats that you should focus on: omega-3 and omega-6 fats. These are known as essential fatty acids, because we need them to function optimally but are unable to produce them in our bodies. We need a balanced amount of omega-3 and omega-6 fats; the ideal ratio is 1:1. In modern diets, we already get more than enough omega-6 fats, so we need to focus on increasing our omega-3 fats while reducing the omega-6 fats found in processed vegetable oils, processed foods, and factory-farmed meats. Some examples of foods rich in omega-3s are hemp seeds, chia seeds, flax seeds, and wild-caught, fatty fish. By eating a diet high in omega-3s, you will be supporting your body's ability to fight inflammation while also protecting your brain and heart health.

Saturated Fats (Short and Medium Chain)

Good saturated fats come from short- and medium-chain fatty acids found in organic butter, egg yolks, coconuts, and grass-fed meats. Short-chain fatty acids are the easiest for the body to convert into energy and can help increase metabolism. Similarly, medium-chain fatty acids are rapidly broken down and absorbed by the body; the highest concentration of these fatty acids is found in coconut oil. Cooking oils that are composed primarily of saturated fats, such as ghee or coconut oil, are solid at room temperature. Saturated fats are the best choice for cooking because they don't oxidize or become damaged when heated. These are the fats our ancestors ate for thousands of years as a source of nourishment.

On Cooking with Good Fat

When cooking, it is essential to know the smoke points of your cooking oils to avoid releasing harmful free radicals into your food. Extra-virgin olive oil isn't recommended for cooking at high temperatures, as it will oxidize, thereby destroying its beneficial properties. On the other hand, ghee is great for cooking at high temperatures because it has the highest smoke point of any unrefined oil. In cases where you need a neutral-flavoured oil, I suggest using naturally refined avocado oil. Avocado oil is one of the only oils that can be refined without chemicals, due to its unique fat composition and unusually high smoke point. Its neutral flavour makes it an excellent substitute for any vegetable oil you normally use for cooking. The following table lists the healthiest oils and fats for cooking, along with their smoke points, storage instructions, and some suggested uses. I haven't included any nut or seed oils, because they contain delicate polyunsaturated fats that should never be heated or used for cooking. Instead, these oils can be used as finishing oils to add flavour to a dish.

Recommended Cooking Oil or Fat	Type of Fat	Smoke Point	Storage Instructions	Shelf Life (After Opening)	Suggested Uses
Avocado oil, naturally refined	Monounsaturated fat	480°F (250°C) High	Store in a cool, dark place	6 months	Frying, roasting, and sautéing when a neutral flavour is desired
Ghee (clarified butter)	Saturated fat	450°F (230°C) High	Store in the fridge or in a cool, dark place	12 months refrigerated, 3 months at room temperature	Frying, sautéing, roasting, and stir frying
Virgin coconut oil	Saturated fat	350°F (180°C) Moderate	Store in a cool, dark place	24 months	Use as a vegan substitute for ghee or when a coconut flavour is desired
Extra-virgin olive oil	Monounsaturated fat	325°F (160°C) Moderate	Store in a cool, dark place	12 months	Low- to medium-heat cooking only, vinaigrettes, finishing oil
Unsalted organic butter	Saturated fat	300°F (150°C) Low	Store in the fridge	3 months	Low-heat cooking only, spreading on bread, melting on pancakes or waffles

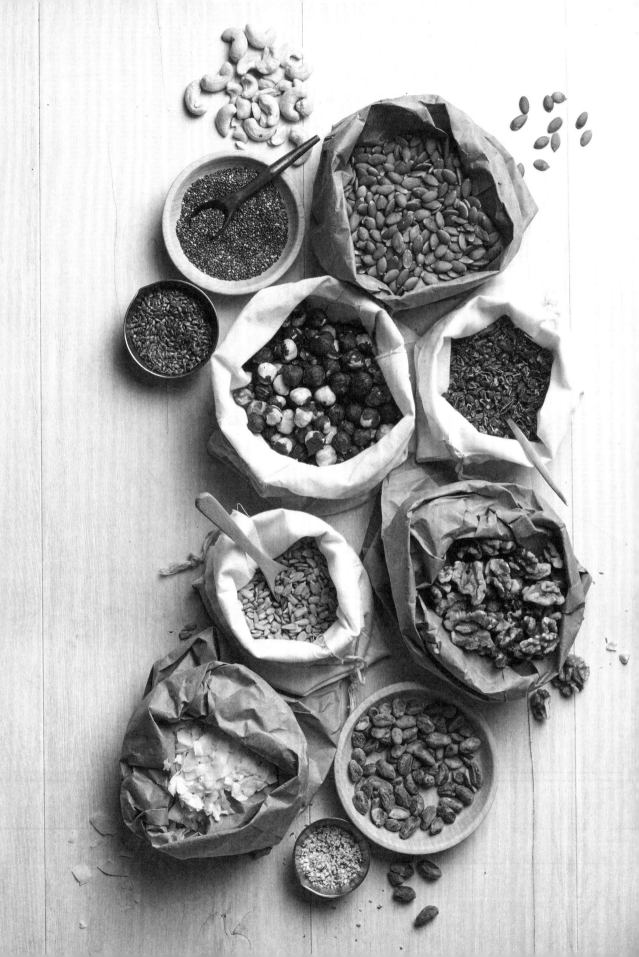

The Fat-Fuelled Pantry

Healthy Fats and Oils

It is essential to use a variety of good fats each day, as each type of fat has different benefits and properties. The fats and oils below are full of goodness and flavour. They form the basis of the recipes in this book, so make sure to stock your pantry full of these healthy sources of fat!

Ghee (Clarified Butter)

Ghee is a type of slow-cooked clarified butter that has a delicious, buttery flavour and a very high smoke point—making it an excellent choice for cooking at high temperatures. Ghee is a source of butyric acid, known to be beneficial for healing the gut, and conjugated linoleic acid (CLA), a fatty acid that may help prevent heart disease. The lactose and milk proteins are removed from the butter, making it easy to digest. If you are shopping at a supermarket, look for ghee that is certified organic to ensure that it does not contain residual antibiotics or pesticides, which accumulate in the milk fat.

In addition, look for ghee that is packaged in glass jars, which prevent plastic chemicals from leaching into the ghee. When made well, ghee is shelf stable and can be kept at room temperature for up to three months or in the fridge for up to twelve months. Always use a clean, dry utensil to dip into the jar and close the lid after each use.

Avocado Oil

Avocado oil has one of the highest smoke points, so it is an excellent choice for high-heat cooking like frying or searing. Due to its unusually high smoke point, avocado oil can be naturally refined without the use of chemicals to give it a neutral flavour. This makes it perfect to use when you do not want to add any flavour to a dish. Avocado oil is high in monounsaturated fats, making it a very healthy oil to have in your pantry. Always purchase avocado oil that has been naturally refined and is in a dark-coloured glass bottle.

Virgin Coconut Oil

Virgin, unrefined coconut oil is another excellent cooking oil due to its relatively high smoke point. Coconut oil is rich in medium-chain fatty acids, which are easy to digest and provide a quick source of energy for the mind and body. Due to its inherent coconut flavour, this oil is best used to enhance the existing coconut flavour of a dish (such as the Tahini-Coconut Fat Balls on page 187). I do not recommend refined coconut oil, because it is usually chemically processed to remove the coconut flavour and scent, which destroys many of its nutritional benefits. Coconut oil is solid at room temperature and turns liquid above 25°C (77°F).

Extra-Virgin Olive Oil (EVOO)

Extra-virgin olive oil is a fantastic source of antioxidants and heart-healthy monounsaturated fats. It is also known to be good for boosting memory and brain function. The mark of good olive oil is a fruity or spicy flavour, which means it is fresh. Unfortunately, many olive oils on the market are adulterated, so it can be hard to find one you can trust. To ensure that you are getting the good stuff, look for olive oil sold in a dark-coloured glass bottle that has a harvest year. Olive oil is not recommended for high-heat cooking and should be used only at low to medium heat or as a finishing oil.

Almond Butter and Tahini

Almond butter and tahini (sesame butter) are a great source of omega-3 fatty acids. I like to use them to drizzle on just about anything. Almond butter is my go-to nut butter, and tahini is my preferred seed butter—I keep a large jar of each in my fridge. They add a nutty flavour, creamy texture, and dose of healthy fats to meals. They can be drizzled on oatmeal, smoothies, roasted vegetables, noodle dishes, and desserts. You can even make your own almond butter (see page 275) if you are so inclined.

Coconut Butter

Coconut butter, also called coconut manna, is made of dried coconut flesh that is ground to a smooth consistency. My favourite ways to use it are in drinks, on toast, or for baking—but it is also delicious eaten straight off a spoon. Coconut butter is found in health food stores, but if you cannot find it, virgin coconut oil will work as a substitute. To drizzle or spread coconut butter, you may need to heat it. Simply place the jar in a hot water bath for 5 to 10 minutes until the coconut butter is softened.

Cacao Butter

Cacao butter, also known as cocoa butter, is a healthy fat derived from unprocessed cocoa beans. It can be found at health food stores and melted to add a rich, chocolatey flavour to baked goods and drinks. I absolutely adore it in my Cacao Butter Hot Chocolate (page 228).

Raw Nuts and Seeds

The recipes in this book always call for raw nuts and seeds. Nuts and seeds are a great source of monounsaturated fats, omega-3 fatty acids, protein, and fibre. Use them to add crunch and staying power to yogurt, granola, oatmeal, and salads. Buying nuts and seeds in bulk is considerably more cost-effective, and many bulk stores will now allow you to bring in your own containers to reduce waste. Just be sure to smell and taste bulk nuts and seeds before you buy them, to check if they have gone rancid. If they are bitter and stale, they are probably past their prime. All nuts and seeds should be kept refrigerated, if possible, to keep them fresh.

Almonds

Almonds are incredibly versatile and can be used to make milk, butter, flour, granola, and snacks. Their unique flavour, allergen-free nature, and health benefits have made them explode in popularity recently. They are high in monounsaturated fats that help balance cholesterol and keep your heart in good shape. Many recipes in this book use almonds in their various forms, so make sure to find a bulk supplier!

Cashews

Cashews are a powerhouse of healthy monounsaturated fats, protein, vitamins, and minerals. When soaked and blended, they add a delicious creamy texture to sauces, soups, and desserts. Soaking cashews also renders them easier to digest, so it is a win-win situation! Raw cashews make a great snack, and I will sometimes fry them in ghee for added flavour and fats.

Pecans

Pecans are higher in fats and lower in carbohydrates than other nuts, making them a perfect option for those who are looking to reduce their carbohydrate intake. Their good fats come from mono-unsaturated and omega-3 fatty acids, which help stabilize hunger and blood sugar while working to keep your heart healthy. They make a delicious snack or crunchy topping on salads and desserts. My favourite way to use them is in the dangerously good Candied Pecans (page 93). Be sure to store pecans in the fridge, as their high fat content makes them more susceptible to rancidity than other nuts.

Hazelnuts

Hazelnuts are a dense source of monoun-saturated fats, along with magnesium and calcium. To bring out their nutty flavour, toast them in a dry skillet for a few minutes and then roughly chop them before adding to salads or desserts. If you are feeling dec-adent, you can substitute toasted hazelnuts for almonds in Homemade Almond Butter (page 275) to make hazelnut butter. Add a pinch of real vanilla powder, and you will have a most delicious treat that you'll eat straight out of the jar.

Pistachios

Pistachios are full of good monounsaturated fats, protein, and fibre. They also contain healthy omega-3 fatty acids that regulate hunger and keep your blood sugar in check. I love eating them by the handful or using them to add colour and crunch to both sweet and savoury dishes. Look for shelled pista-chios that are whole, raw, and unsalted. Unshelled is fine, too, if you have time on your hands. They are the star of the show in my Maple Pistachio Baklava (page 239).

Macadamia Nuts

Macadamias are prized for their creamy texture and buttery flavour. Their flavour comes from the fact that they have the highest amount of monounsaturated fat and the lowest amounts of carbohydrates, fibre, and protein when compared to other nuts. For this reason, macadamia nuts are another great option for those on low-carb diets. They can be ground to a coarse meal and used as a substitute in any recipe that calls for bread crumbs. I love snacking on raw macadamia nuts and using them to make macadamia milk (see page 273) for a decadently creamy, dairy-free milk alternative. Although I love macadamia nuts, they are quite expensive, so I do not use them often.

Walnuts

Walnuts are one of the healthiest nuts you can eat. They are often referred to as brain food because they are very high in omega-3 fatty acids, monounsaturated fats, and antioxidants. Their high fibre content also helps regulate cholesterol levels. They make a great snack or addition to Grainless Ghee-nola (page 52). The combination of protein, healthy fats, and fibre in walnuts will keep you satisfied.

Pumpkin Seeds

Also known as pepitas, pumpkin seeds are a powerhouse of nutrition, as they contain valuable minerals such as magnesium, manganese, and zinc in addition to heart-healthy fats. I love munching on them raw as a snack, adding them to salads, and incorporating them into baked goods. If you can find the dark green Styrian pumpkin seeds, they are higher in antioxidants (and more delicious) than the common pumpkin seed variety.

Sunflower Seeds

Sunflower seeds are rich in healthy fats and can help keep your appetite regular. They are also a great source of antioxidants that reduce inflammation and help protect the body from free radical damage. I add sunflower seeds to a bowl of trail mix that I keep on my kitchen counter for snacking throughout the day. They are also great to sprinkle on salads for some extra crunch. Sunflower seeds are inexpensive, so you are getting good bang for your buck!

Sesame Seeds

Sesame seeds are a dense source of healthy fats, fibre, and protein. Like most other nuts and seeds, sesame seeds are very prone to rancidity, so it is best to purchase them raw and keep them in the refrigerator until you are ready to use them. Before using, simply toast them in a dry skillet for a few minutes until they are fragrant and golden brown. Sprinkle them on soups, salads, grain bowls, salmon, and desserts for an earthy, nutty flavour. Sesame seeds can be ground into tahini, a versatile nut-free butter used for cooking and baking.

Flax Seeds

Flax seeds are one of the healthiest seeds you can buy. They are known for having among the highest levels of omega-3 fatty acids and fibre of any seed (alongside chia and hemp seeds). To get the most benefit from flax seeds, purchase them whole and store them in the fridge until you are ready to use them. Before using, grind them into meal using a coffee grinder or a mortar and pestle. Stay away from pre-ground flax seeds and flaxseed oil, which are highly oxidized and have little nutritional value remaining.

Chia Seeds

Chia seeds are small but mighty—they were prized by the Aztecs as a source of energy and strength. Although chia seeds are similar to flax seeds in terms of their very high omega-3 ratio, they do not go rancid as quickly and can be stored at room temperature. To activate chia seeds and maximize their benefits, add them to any liquid, such as yogurt, coconut milk, or smoothies, and let them soak for 10 to 15 minutes. My favourite way to use them is in Watermelon Chia Fresca (page 219), which is super refreshing in the summer.

Hemp Seeds

Hemp seeds are a great source of plant-based protein, as they contain all nine essential amino acids. Hemp seeds should always be kept refrigerated to prevent rancidity; however, unlike flax and chia seeds, they do not need to be soaked or ground before use. This makes them easy to sprinkle on just about anything, such as oatmeal, toast, or salads. I like blending a tablespoon or two of hemp seeds into my smoothie for protein and heart-healthy omega-3 fatty acids.

Dried Coconut

Dried coconut comes in two forms: flakes and shredded. Coconut flakes are different from shredded coconut and come in large pieces that are great to use as a crunchy topper or to make Raw Chipotle Spiced Coconut Chips (page 188). Both forms of dried coconut are a great source of medium-chain triglycerides (MCTs), which provide a quick source of energy for your mind and body. The recipes in this book call for unsweetened coconut to avoid added sugars.

Acids and Vinegar

Using acids and vinegar is especially crucial in dishes that contain a lot of healthy fats. They work to cut through all the richness and balance out the flavours. A little acidity goes a long way—often just a single tablespoon of apple cider vinegar or lemon juice is enough to round out a dish and take it to a whole new level.

Raw Apple Cider Vinegar

Apple cider vinegar, or "ACV," is the healthiest vinegar you can buy. I use it in salad dressings and whenever I need a touch of acidity to balance a recipe. Notice how a splash of vinegar really helps the flavours pop in my Creamy Tomato Soup with Garlic Sourdough Croutons (page 80) or Sheet Pan Sausage Dinner with Caramelized Cabbage and Red Onion (page 140). Look for organic, raw, and unfiltered apple cider vinegar "with the mother." The mother is the beneficial bacteria that ferment the apple juice into vinegar.

Balsamic Vinegar and Balsamic Reduction

An excellent balsamic vinegar is a treasure to behold, and much like olive oil, its quality is super important. Look for the words "balsamic vinegar of Modena" and check the ingredients list to ensure that there are no added sulphites (naturally occurring sulphites will not be listed in the ingredients). I also love to use balsamic reductions in cooking; these can be made at home by simmering balsamic vinegar until it reduces to a thick, syrupy consistency. They are great for drizzling on salads as well as my Bone Broth Braised Leek and Goat Cheese Galette (page 169).

Lemons and Limes

Fresh lemons and limes are pantry essentials. They are great to have on hand for making freshly squeezed juice on a moment's notice. I recommend buying them by the bag to make sure you always have some ready for adding brightness to the recipes in this book. Make sure to get them organic, so that you can grate the zest or use the lemon whole, without having to worry about pesticide residues leaching into your food.

Full-Fat Dairy, Eggs, and Smoked Fish

Studies have shown that those who eat full-fat dairy tend to have lower rates of obesity-related disease. Always buy full-fat dairy products made from organic, unhomogenized milk—preferably from goat's or sheep's milk, as these are easier for the body to break down. Here are some of my favourite dairy products, eggs, and smoked fish.

Goat Cheese

Goat cheese is one of the healthiest cheeses you can buy. It is an exceptional source of healthy fats like medium-chain fatty acids, which provide a quick source of energy for the mind and body. Although the amount of fat in goat cheese is similar to that in cow's milk cheeses, the different protein structure in goat cheese makes it easier to digest. I often use goat cheese in salads, and it adds a delightfully tangy flavour to my Cardamom Date Cake with Goat Cheese Frosting (page 255).

Pecorino Romano

Pecorino Romano is a hard cheese made from raw sheep's milk. As with all hard cheeses, most of the lactose is removed, which makes it very easy to digest. I use Pecorino in many of the recipes in this book, so it is worth seeking out in the cheese section at your local grocery store. You can also use Parmesan cheese in place of Pecorino; it has a milder flavour and is made from raw cow's milk rather than sheep's milk. In addition to being rich sources of healthy fats, hard cheeses are also excellent sources of protein.

Goat's and Sheep's Milk Feta

Feta is traditionally made from sheep's or goat's milk; however, in North America, most feta cheese is made from pasteurized cow's milk. I prefer the traditional goat's or sheep's milk varieties, as they are easier to digest and have a creamier texture. You can find them at cheese shops, farmers markets, or specialty food stores.

Halloumi

Similar to feta, halloumi cheese is traditionally made from sheep's milk, but nowadays it is usually made from cow's milk. Sheep's milk halloumi is preferred but is harder to find. Look for it at cheese shops, farmers markets, or specialty stores. Halloumi has a high melting point, which means you can fry it until it turns golden without the cheese melting. Serve fried halloumi as a tasty, fat-fuelled appetizer, or use it in my Warm Quinoa Salad with Fried Halloumi and Bacon (page 98).

Organic or Grass-Fed Plain Full-Fat Yogurt

If you can tolerate dairy, plain full-fat yogurt is a great thing to include in your diet. It contains a lot of healthy saturated fats, omega-3 fatty acids, vitamins, protein, and probiotics. Full-fat yogurt can come from cow's, sheep's, buffalo, or goat's milk. Each variety has a distinct flavour, and all of them can be found in the natural section of a well-stocked grocery store. I buy the ones that come in a glass jar and have a thick layer of cream on top, which I like to scoop off and eat with a spoon.

Organic or Grass-Fed Butter

Organic or grass-fed butter is a dense source of fat-soluble vitamins and healthy fats. I suggest buying some and using it to make a batch of ghee, as it lasts longer and can be used for cooking at higher temperatures (see page 271).

Pasture-Raised Eggs or Organic

When it comes to eggs, look for ones that are preferably pasture-raised, which means the chickens were able to roam freely outdoors and forage on their natural diet. This allows them to produce eggs with bright orange yolks—a signifier of high Vitamin A and omega-3 fatty acid content. In a pinch, organic eggs will do the trick too. Unless otherwise specified, all the recipes in this book call for large eggs.

Smoked Sockeye Salmon

Salmon is high in vitamin D, which is essential for nutrient absorption. You can buy it frozen and store it in your freezer. Defrost it any time you want to add healthy fats and protein to grain bowls, eggs, and toast. Look for the sockeye variety, which has a vibrant red flesh. Sockeye contains a lot of healthy omega-3 fatty acids, which are linked to better memory. Since sockeye is always wild-caught, you avoid the harmful dyes and antibiotics found in farmed salmon.

Smoked Trout

My favourite way to use smoked trout is to make it into a spread and smear it on Grain-Free Everything Bagels (page 67). It is also delicious flaked into salads like my Black Kale Salad with Smoked Trout and Hazelnuts (page 110) for added protein and omega-3 fatty acids. Be sure to buy smoked trout from a reputable fishmonger, as the quality makes all the difference in flavour. The fat in smoked trout is the good kind, so feel free to enjoy it often!

Flours

There are many healthier alternatives to all-purpose white flour that work just as well, if not better! I love to experiment and use a variety of them to take advantage of their unique baking properties and nutrients.

Sprouted or Light Spelt Flour

Sprouted spelt flour is a staple in my pantry. Light spelt flour can be substituted, but sprouted spelt flour is more easily digested. I always keep it on hand for cooking and baking due to its versatility and neutral taste. Although the gluten in spelt flour is easier to digest than that in wheat flour, you can substitute the same quantity of gluten-free all-purpose flour or cassava flour to yield similar results.

Gluten-Free All-Purpose Flour

Gluten-free all-purpose flour is an alternative to sprouted and light spelt flour for those who are gluten intolerant. You can find 1:1 gluten-free all-purpose flour at health food stores or in the natural section of a well-stocked grocery store. Other gluten-free flours such as chickpea flour and buckwheat flour will not yield the same results in recipes that call for gluten-free all-purpose flour, so reserve them for recipes that call for those specific varieties.

Cassava Flour

Cassava flour is a grain-free flour derived from the cassava root, and an equal amount of cassava flour can be substituted in recipes that call for sprouted or light spelt flour. Tapioca flour is also derived from the cassava root, but the flours are quite different and cannot be used interchangeably. Cassava flour can be found in health food stores or easily be purchased online. The brand of cassava flour you use can vary in terms of quality and taste. I used Otto's Naturals Cassava Flour to make the recipes in this book.

Super-Fine Blanched Almond Flour

Blanched almond flour is ground from skinless, whole almonds. It adds a delicate texture to baked goods and contains a lot of good fats, fibre, and protein. It is incredibly nutritious, and I recommend getting it from bulk stores to stock your pantry for baking and cooking. I absolutely love using blanched almond flour to make my Crispy Almond Flour Waffles with Coconut Whipped Cream (page 48)!

Coconut Flour

Coconut flour is ground from dried coconut meat. It is a delicious nut-free, grain-free flour alternative. Just like almond flour, it is high in fibre, protein, and healthy fats. You cannot substitute coconut flour for other flours in a 1:1 ratio, so it is best used only when called for in a recipe.

Arrowroot Starch

I use arrowroot starch as a cornstarch replacement to thicken soups, stews, and gravies. It is GMO-free and processed without the use of harsh chemicals, making it a healthier option. It can be found at bulk stores and health food stores or in the natural section of a well-stocked grocery store. If you prefer to use cornstarch, you can substitute it at a ratio of 3:2—1 tablespoon (15 mL) of cornstarch to 2 teaspoons (10 mL) of arrowroot starch.

Natural Sweeteners

There seem to be millions of natural sweeteners on the market, with new ones popping up every day. I am skeptical of anything that wasn't around when my grandparents were young and prefer unprocessed, natural sweeteners like raw honey and maple syrup. When you cook or bake with natural sweeteners, it is essential to include healthy fats and fibre, which help balance blood sugar.

Pure Maple Syrup

Given my Canadian background, it is no surprise that maple syrup is my favourite natural sweetener. In addition to its lovely caramel taste, it has the benefits of containing trace minerals and vitamins. I usually opt for dark maple syrup and get it in large 2-quart (2 L) jugs from the farmers market. Always store maple syrup in the fridge, to prevent it from going mouldy.

Raw Honey

Honey is a delicious sweetener that is slightly sweeter than maple syrup. According to Ayurveda, heating honey can change its chemical structure and make it lose its essential enzymes and nutrients. For this reason, I do not suggest using it in cooking or baking when direct heat is involved. Always look for raw honey that is local and unpasteurized to get the maximum health benefits it can offer.

Medjool Dates

Dates are a great source of fibre and potassium. I use them to create the moist texture in my Cardamom Date Cake with Goat Cheese Frosting (page 255). Look for very soft Medjool dates. This means they are fresh and will blend effortlessly into smoothies, batters, and doughs. My favourite fat-fuelled snack is a Medjool date stuffed with ghee, almond butter, and pistachios.

Coconut Sugar

Coconut sugar is made from dried coconut palm sap. I love the rich, molasses-like taste and use it in baked goods wherever a granulated sugar is needed. It is a healthier, less processed alternative to white or brown sugar. You can find coconut sugar in the sugar aisle of any well-stocked grocery store.

Dark Chocolate

Dark chocolate is a surprisingly dense source of healthy fats, antioxidants, and magnesium. The good fat in chocolate comes from cacao butter, which is derived from cacao beans. I always keep some dark chocolate on hand for baking my Molten Chocolate Lava Cakes (page 256) and for snacking! Look for dark chocolate that is 70 percent cacao or higher.

Canned Goods and Condiments

These are the canned, jarred, and bottled items that I always have stocked in my pantry for cooking and baking. Many of them are common ingredients, whereas a couple of them require a trip to a specialty food store.

Canned Full-Fat Coconut Milk

I always have a few cans of full-fat coconut milk on hand. I often use it to add creaminess to dishes, instead of using heavy cream. It is essential to find a brand that does not contain any additives; the only two ingredients should be coconut extract and water. Aroy-D is a widely available brand that meets all the criteria above, is very inexpensive, and tastes great!

Canned Coconut Cream

Coconut cream is not the same as creamed coconut. It comes in a can and can be found at health food stores. To make it at home, simply refrigerate a can of full-fat coconut milk overnight. Scoop out the thick layer of cream on top and use it to add extra richness to dairy-free dishes and to make Coconut Whipped Cream (page 274).

Canned Tomatoes and Tomato Paste

Look for tomatoes and tomato paste in glass jars, as the acidity from tomatoes in metal cans can cause the lining to break down and leach chemicals. I like the brand Bioitalia, which has a line of organic tomatoes in glass jars. Whole canned tomatoes have a lot more flavour than crushed ones. If you have time, you can buy whole canned tomatoes and crush them yourself to use in recipes that call for crushed tomatoes.

Canned Sockeye Salmon

Canned sockeye salmon is an inexpensive source of omega-3 fatty acids, vitamin D, and protein. I always have a few cans of sockeye salmon on hand, to eat as a snack or add to salads. I recommend sockeye salmon because it is wild-caught and contains more omega-3s than farmed salmon. Always look for canned salmon with the bones and skin. The skin contains much of the omega-3 fatty acids, and the bones are a great source of calcium, which strengthens bones and teeth.

Canned Beans

Canned beans are great to have on hand for making simple vegetarian dishes. I recommend using the Eden Organic brand because they soak their beans overnight and cook them with kombu seaweed. This makes them easier to digest and reduces bloating. For time-saving reasons, the recipes in this book mainly call for canned beans; however, you are more than welcome to soak dried beans overnight and cook them.

Organic Chicken and Beef Broth

Using a high-quality broth is the secret to making dishes flavourful and nutrient dense. Of course, it is always best to use homemade Bone Broth (page 272), but for those times when you are in a pinch, it is useful to have a few Tetra Paks of organic chicken and beef broth in your pantry. The recipes in this book call for seasoned broth, so make sure to avoid low-sodium varieties. Look for brands that season with sea salt and buy organic, if possible.

Gluten-Free Tamari

Gluten-free tamari is a type of soy sauce made without wheat or gluten. If you cannot eat soy, coconut aminos seasoning is a great alternative made from fermented coconut sap. It has a similar flavour and is suitable for a variety of dietary restrictions and food sensitivities. Although it is referred to as coconut aminos in the United States, it goes by soy-free seasoning sauce in Canada.

Pomegranate Molasses

Pomegranate molasses adds a tangy, sweet, and sharp flavour to Middle Eastern–inspired dishes. I always have it in my fridge and use it often in meat dishes, braises, and stews. It is a key ingredient in my Pistachio-Crusted Rack of Lamb with Pomegranate Butter Glaze (page 139). You can find pomegranate molasses at specialty food stores, or you can make it at home by simmering pomegranate juice until it reduces to a thick, syrupy consistency.

Harissa Paste

Harissa paste is a delicious North African chili paste. I really like the brand Belazu, which I have used in creating many of the recipes in this book. It comes in a glass jar and can be found online or at specialty food stores. Different brands of harissa paste vary significantly in their spice levels. If you are using another brand, you may want to add more or less harissa paste, depending on the level of spiciness you want to achieve.

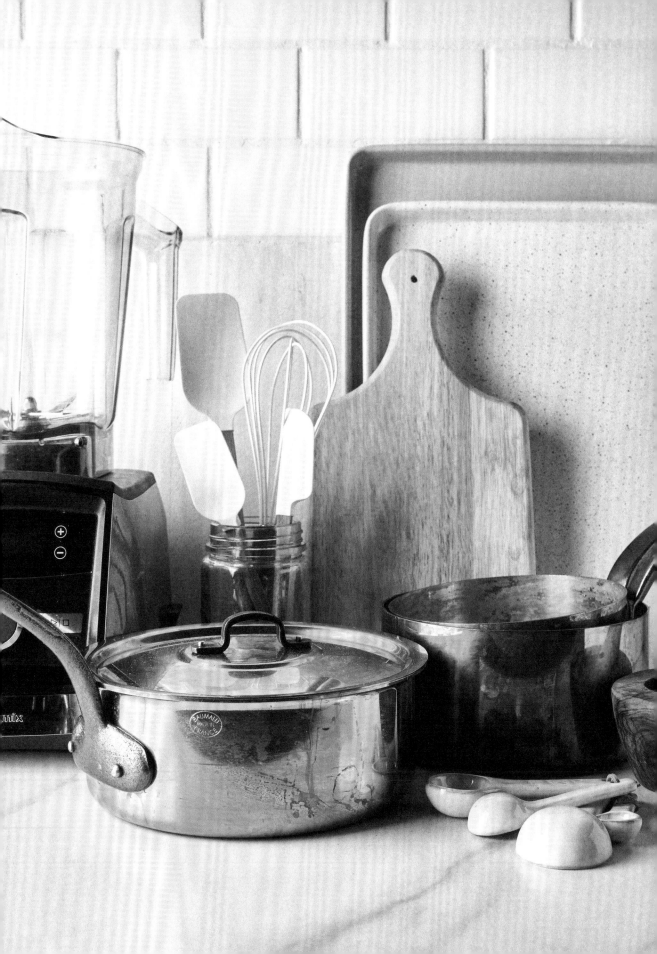

Tools and Equipment

Every craft requires a set of tools and equipment. I started my cooking journey in my early twenties with limited kitchen tools—a hot plate and a toaster oven, to be precise. Over time I have added all the essential cooking tools and some splurge-worthy items that I treasure. Once I got to the point in life where I could afford to invest in higher quality things, I opted for appliances that do not break after a handful of uses. I learned that this can actually save you money in the long run, as these items often last a lifetime. Each new piece opened up a world of possibilities in the kitchen and made me a better cook as a result. Here, I have outlined the tools and equipment you need to make the recipes in this book successfully and with ease.

Small Tools

- Measuring cups
- Measuring spoons
- Box grater
- Whisks
- Wooden spoons
- Spatulas
- Chef's knife
- Fine mesh strainer

Tools for the Stove and Oven

Medium 10-inch (25 cm) and large 12-inch (30 cm) Cast-Iron Skillets

Cast-iron skillets are inexpensive, durable, heat-safe, and oven-safe. If you do not own a set, buy one now. It will be one of the best investments you will ever make. These skillets last a lifetime and can be used for just about anything, from frying on the stovetop to broiling in the oven.

Good-Quality Nonstick Pan

Having a good-quality nonstick pan is useful for making scrambled eggs or pancakes, which usually like to stick to the pan. Unlike cast-iron skillets, nonstick pans should never be used for cooking above medium temperatures. Look for nonstick pans that are nontoxic, ceramic coated, and free of harmful chemicals and heavy metals.

2-Quart (2 L) Saucepan

I use a variety of saucepans that range from 1 quart (1 L) to 4 quarts (4 L); however, the only saucepan you really need is a medium 2-quart (2 L) saucepan with a lid. You can use this standard size for most cooking purposes. If a large saucepan is called for in a recipe and you don't have one, a stock pot will work just as well.

6-Quart (6 L) Large Dutch Oven

A large, enamel-coated Dutch oven or other heavy-bottomed pot with a tight-fitting lid is the perfect vessel to slow-cook stews and braises. It has fantastic heat transferability and can be placed both on the stovetop and in the oven. It is also great for browning and shallow frying because the sides are deep enough to avoid making a mess.

Stock Pot

A stock pot is necessary for making large batches of Bone Broth (page 272), which forms the base of many recipes in this book. I also pull out my stock pot for boiling potatoes or pasta.

Baking Dishes

For baking, you will need a variety of dishes. Depending on the material of your baking dishes, the cooking time may vary slightly. I have made the recipes in this book using glass or light-coloured ceramic baking dishes, so if you use a dark-coloured baking dish, you may need to lower your oven temperature slightly. If you are using shiny metal baking dishes, these may cause the food to bake slower and need a bit more time in the oven. The recipes call for a glass 8-inch (2 L) square baking dish, in addition to 11- × 7-inch (2 L) and 12½- × 8½-inch (3.5 L) baking dishes.

Loaf Pan
I occasionally use a 9- × 5-inch (2 L) loaf pan for baking loaf cakes and bread. Like baking dishes, different coloured loaf pans conduct heat differently. For consistent results, I recommend using a loaf pan that is made from dark metal. If you are using a shiny metal loaf pan, it may cause the food to bake slower and need a bit more time in the oven.

Half Sheet Pan
The standard-size baking sheet for home ovens is called a half sheet pan and measures 18 × 13 inches (45 × 33 cm), with sides about 1 inch (2.5 cm) high. For several years, I had a tiny oven that couldn't fit a standard half sheet pan. I had to use quarter baking sheets and make things in several batches or go over to my mother's house to use her oven. Although the recipes mainly call for standard half sheet pans, I will occasionally turn to my trusty quarter baking sheets to make things easier when I am roasting things separately at the same time.

Appliances

14-Cup Food Processor
I use my food processor for many purposes, such as making nut flours, spelt pastry dough, cake batters, sourdough bread crumbs, sauces, chutneys, nut butter, dips, pesto, and aioli. I have gone through many food processors, but my favourite is my Cuisinart, which has a powerful motor. A mini food processor is not necessary but comes in handy for smaller jobs, such as making only ½ cup (125 mL) of oat flour for the Easy Banana Oat Pancakes (page 47).

High-Speed Blender
A handful of recipes in this book call for a high-speed blender. A high-speed blender has a strong motor and can do things for which a regular blender is not powerful enough. This is important for recipes that have tougher ingredients like frozen fruit, nuts, and dates, to achieve a smooth consistency. If you use a regular blender, the results may vary.

Electric Beaters

I do not bake often, so I don't own a stand mixer. Instead, I use my trusty electric beaters, which can perform many of the same kitchen tasks. I whip them out occasionally for beating egg whites or if I am making a batch of Coconut Whipped Cream (page 274). Of course, you can always use a hand whisk (and some elbow grease) if you do not own electric beaters.

Waffle Iron

A waffle iron will help you take your weekend brunches to another level. Quality does make a difference, and some waffle irons are better than others. I have a Hamilton Beach Belgian-style waffle maker, and I think it is the bee's knees. If you can borrow one from a friend or a family member, that works too.

Microplane Grater

A Microplane grater is a life-changing instrument used for finely grating ingredients like lemon zest, dark chocolate, hard cheeses, whole spices, garlic, and ginger. My favourite way to use it is to finely grate garlic for salad dressings. As a bonus, if you happen to burn a piece of toast, you can use a Microplane grater to shave off those burnt edges. This is a nice-to-have item, not a necessity.

Digital Kitchen Scale

A small digital kitchen scale is a great tool to have for precisely measuring ingredients such as meats and cheeses by weight.

| Extras

Glass Food Storage Containers

Glass food storage containers are safer than plastic containers and are more environmentally friendly. They are great for storing cooked ingredients from meal prep or packing up leftovers. Tempered glass containers can also be used in the oven (without the lid) or in the freezer, and they will not break. Glass mason jars are also great to have on hand for storing nuts, seeds, and flours that you purchase in bulk.

Reusable Silicone Food Storage Bags

Silicone food storage bags are a safer and more environmentally friendly alternative to plastic ones. I use mine for packing snacks to take with me to work, storing prepared ingredients, or freezing food for weeks on end.

Beeswax Wrap

Beeswax wrap is a great invention that can be used in place of plastic wrap as a more environmentally friendly option. Many companies make beeswax wrap these days—it can be used for wrapping up half a lemon or avocado, wrapping cheese, and much more.

Unbleached Cheesecloth

Cheesecloth is essential for making ghee (clarified butter), poaching fish, and straining bone broth. Look for a cheesecloth that has a fine-weave fabric to ensure that nothing slips through, or double it up for extra protection.

Nut Milk Bag

Nut milk is an excellent replacement for regular milk that can be used in cooking, baking, smoothies, and lattes. Making nut milk at home is a great way to save money, and the result is a much tastier, healthier product than you can buy in stores. It is easiest to make nut milk using a nut milk bag, but if you do not have one, you can use cheesecloth or a fine mesh strainer.

Parchment Paper

Parchment paper is great to have on hand for when you want to prevent things from sticking to the pan. Recipes in this book will specify if parchment paper is required. However, if you have aluminum baking sheets, it's best to always use parchment paper, as it creates a barrier to prevent the aluminum from leaching into your food. I use unbleached parchment paper, which is untreated and chlorine-free.

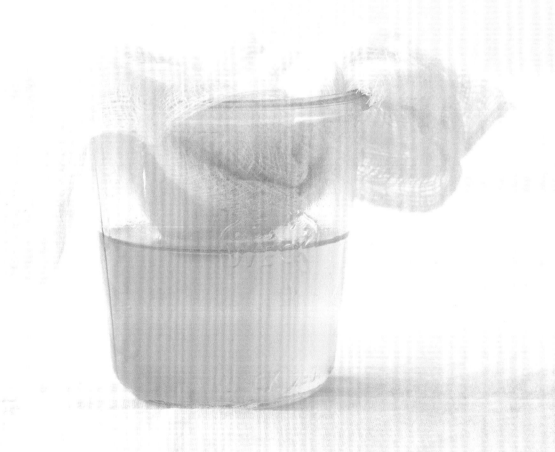

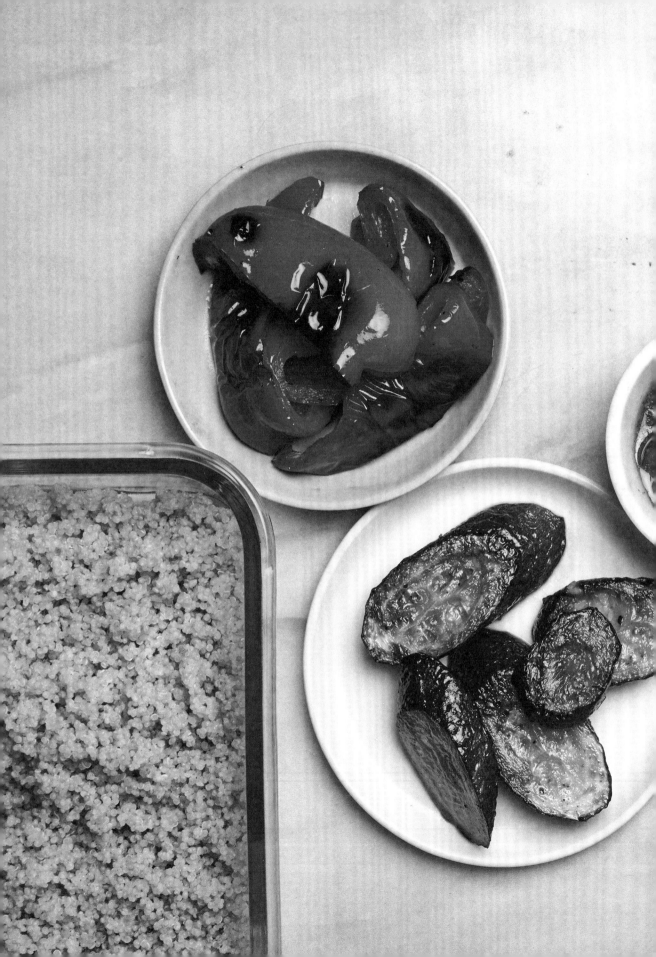

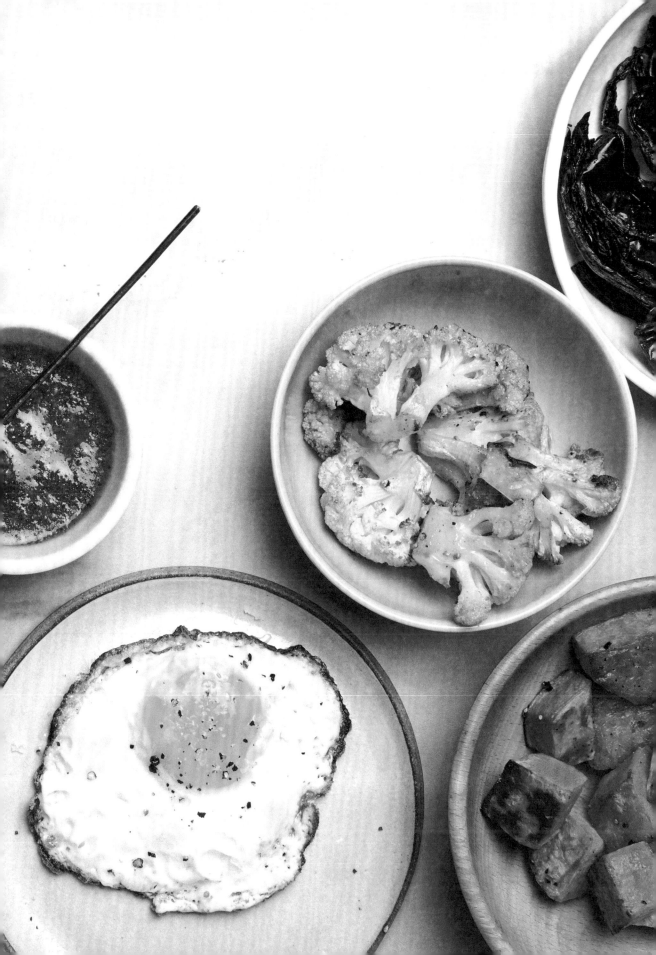

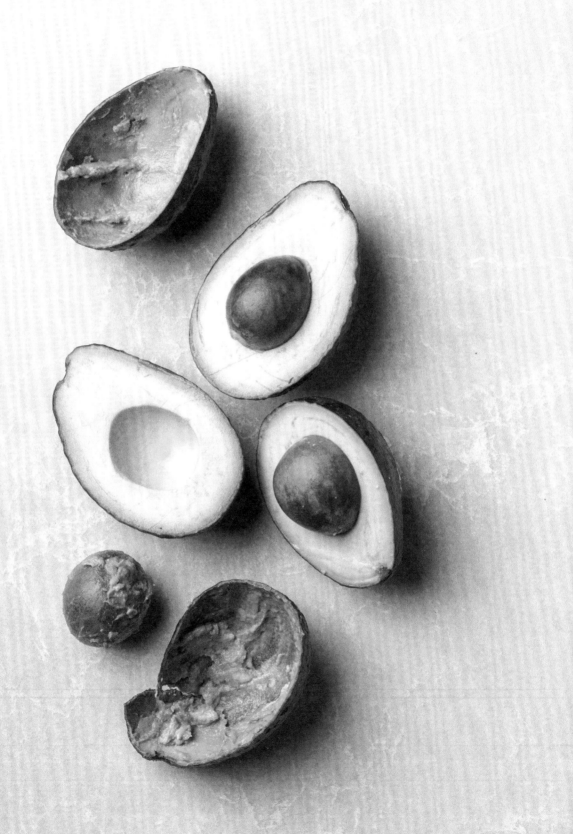

Morning
Eats

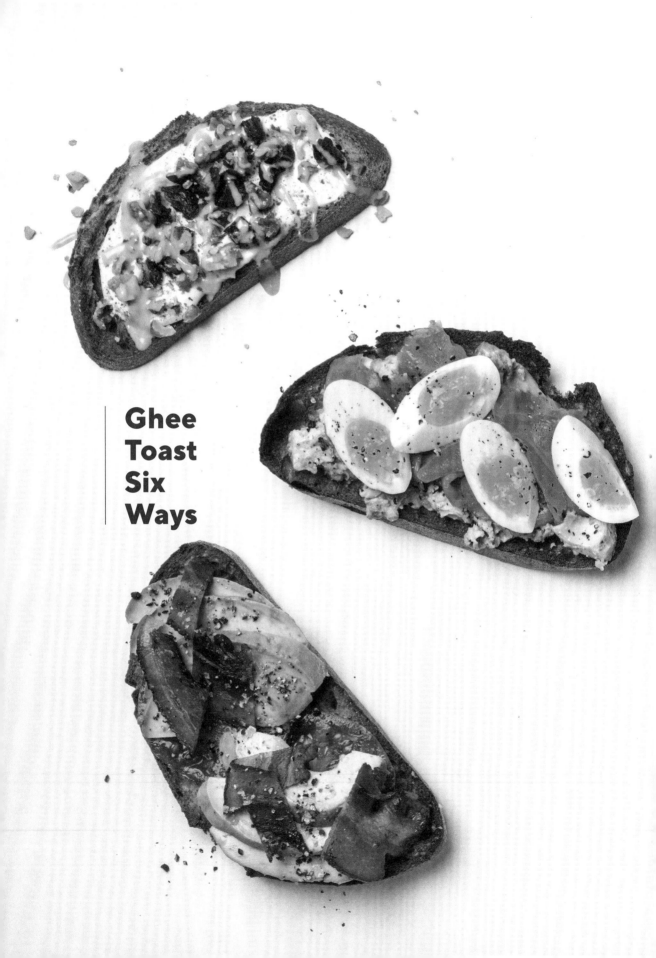

Ghee
Toast
Six
Ways

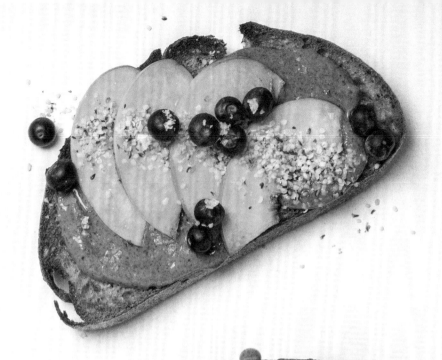

Growing up, I could only eat toast if it was slathered with a lot of butter. As I got older, ghee replaced my butter addiction and became my new favourite toast condiment. Ghee is naturally shelf stable at room temperature, which makes it inherently spreadable. It also tastes incredibly buttery and delicious. Here are some sweet and savoury ghee toasts that I like to make in the morning for breakfast or as a mid-afternoon snack. They are topped with satiating ingredients like nuts and seeds, smoked salmon, Jammy Eggs (page 269), and avocado.

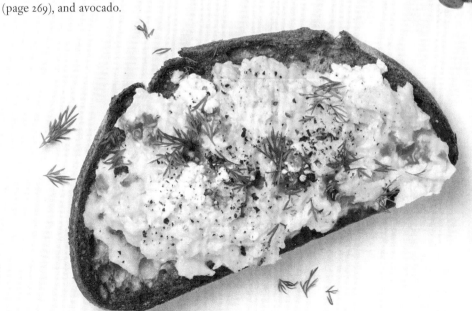

Dates, Walnuts, and Tahini

This ghee toast has an exciting combination of flavours and textures. Between the crunchy walnuts, sweet dates, nutty tahini, and tangy yogurt, each bite is an adventure. The flaky sea salt adds a sweet-and-salty element. A sprinkle makes all the difference, so it's definitely worth having in your pantry.

1 large or 2 small slices of sourdough or gluten-free bread

1 to 2 teaspoons (5 to 10 mL) ghee or Plain Jane Ghee (page 271), at room temperature

1 to 2 tablespoons (15 to 30 mL) plain coconut yogurt or plain full-fat yogurt

Pinch of cinnamon

1 soft Medjool date, pitted and chopped

2 tablespoons (30 mL) chopped raw walnuts

Tahini, to drizzle

Pinch of flaky sea salt (optional)

1. Toast the bread and place it on a plate. Spread the toast with ghee.
2. Top with a layer of yogurt, followed by a sprinkle of cinnamon and the chopped dates and walnuts.
3. Drizzle the tahini on top and finish with a sprinkle of salt, if using.

◆ **Gluten-Free:** Use gluten-free bread instead of sourdough bread. **Dairy-Free:** Use coconut yogurt.

◆ Avocado, Smoked Salmon, and Jammy Egg

An avocado toast to trump all avocado toasts! This recipe uses ghee for a buttery, spreadable base and incorporates healthy fats and protein from smoked salmon and a Jammy Egg. You can make a batch of Jammy Eggs (page 269) ahead of time and store them in the refrigerator for up to 3 days, until you are ready to use them. This toast provides the necessary trifecta of good fats, protein, and carbohydrates that will keep you satisfied for hours. Trust me, it is delicious.

1 large or 2 small slices of sourdough or gluten-free bread

1 to 2 teaspoons (5 to 10 mL) ghee or Plain Jane Ghee (page 271), at room temperature

¼ to ½ avocado, peeled, pitted, and sliced

1 piece of smoked sockeye salmon

1 Jammy Egg (page 269), cut into quarters

Pinch of flaky sea salt (optional)

Freshly ground black pepper

1. Toast the bread and place it on a plate. Spread the toast with ghee.
2. Fan out the avocado slices on top. Using a fork, mash the avocado into the toast.
3. Top with the smoked salmon and pieces of egg.
4. Finish with a sprinkle of salt (if using) and pepper.

◆ **Gluten-Free:** Use gluten-free bread instead of sourdough bread.

◆ Bacon, Avocado, and Tomato

This fat-fuelled version of a classic BLT uses avocado instead of lettuce, which makes it feel more like breakfast. I love the simplicity of ghee toast with sliced tomato, avocado, or bacon by themselves, but the combination of all three together is just heavenly! I suggest making a batch of Perfect Oven Bacon (page 270) during your weekly meal prep and having it on hand for this toast when those hunger cravings hit.

1 large or 2 small slices of sourdough or gluten-free bread

1 to 2 teaspoons (5 to 10 mL) ghee or Plain Jane Ghee (page 271), at room temperature

1 to 2 slices of tomato

¼ to ½ avocado, peeled, pitted, and sliced

1 to 2 slices of Perfect Oven Bacon (page 270), cut into bite-size pieces

1. Toast the bread and place it on a plate. Spread the toast with ghee.

2. Add the tomato, then fan out the avocado slices on top.

3. Top with the bacon pieces.

◆ **Gluten-Free:** Use gluten-free bread instead of sourdough bread.

Ricotta and Smashed Raspberries

This recipe was inspired by the famous ricotta toast at Sqirl in Los Angeles. I don't have a lot of time in the mornings, so I created my own version that is quick to make and includes a lot of healthy fats. Since I don't buy sugary jams anymore, I make an instant chia jam by smashing raspberries with chia seeds—no cooking required. The jam tastes so fruity and delicious that you won't even know it is super good for you!

¼ cup (60 mL) fresh raspberries

½ teaspoon (2 mL) chia seeds

1 large or 2 small slices of sourdough or gluten-free bread

1 to 2 teaspoons (5 to 10 mL) ghee or Plain Jane Ghee (page 271), at room temperature

1 to 2 tablespoons (15 to 30 mL) sheep's milk ricotta cheese

1 tablespoon (15 mL) Grainless Ghee-nola (page 52)

Natural almond butter or Homemade Almond Butter (page 275), to drizzle (optional)

1. In a small bowl, smash together the raspberries and chia seeds with a fork.
2. Toast the bread and place it on a plate. Spread the toast with ghee.
3. Spoon the ricotta on top, spreading it from the centre outward. Top with the chia jam and Grainless Ghee-nola. Drizzle the almond butter on top, if using.

◆ **Gluten-Free:** Use gluten-free bread instead of sourdough bread.

◆ Almond Butter and Peaches

When peach season comes around, I look for any excuse to eat them! This ghee toast topped with almond butter and peaches is one of my favourite ways to take advantage of the summer harvest. The peaches add a juicy, colourful element to an otherwise dry-ish brown toast and truly make your taste buds sing! If peaches are not in season, you can top the toast with blueberries, raspberries, or sliced bananas.

1 large or 2 small slices of sourdough or gluten-free bread

1 to 2 teaspoons (5 to 10 mL) ghee or Plain Jane Ghee (page 271), at room temperature

2 tablespoons (30 mL) natural almond butter or Homemade Almond Butter (page 275)

Pinch of ground cardamom

1 firm-ripe peach, pitted and sliced

Fresh blueberries (optional)

½ teaspoon (2 mL) hemp seeds

1. Toast the bread and place it on a plate. Spread the toast with ghee and then with almond butter.

2. Sprinkle with cardamom. Fan out the peach slices on top and add the blueberries, if using. Finish with a sprinkle of hemp seeds.

◆ **Gluten-Free:** Use gluten-free bread instead of sourdough bread.
Nut-Free: Use sunflower seed butter instead of almond butter.

Soft Scrambled Eggs

I first had soft scrambled eggs with goat cheese while on vacation in the Eastern Townships of Quebec, and now I cannot make them any other way. The goat cheese adds a delightful tangy flavour and creaminess that pairs perfectly with the soft, buttery eggs. Be sure to use a good nonstick pan for this recipe, as it helps the eggs move around freely to form delicate folds.

4 pasture-raised or organic eggs

2 tablespoons (30 mL) water

Pinch of sea salt

1 tablespoon (15 mL) ghee or Plain Jane Ghee (page 271), at room temperature, divided

3 tablespoons (45 mL) crumbled goat cheese

2 large or 4 small slices of sourdough or gluten-free bread

Freshly ground black pepper

1. In a medium bowl, whisk together the eggs, water, and salt until frothy.

2. In a medium nonstick pan over medium heat, melt 1 teaspoon (5 mL) of the ghee. Pour the eggs into the centre of the pan and leave undisturbed for 1 to 2 minutes until the eggs begin to set. Using a spatula, gently push the eggs from the edge of the pan toward the centre. Continue cooking for 1 to 2 minutes, pushing the eggs toward the centre of the pan occasionally and tilting the pan slightly to allow the liquid eggs to fill in the gaps until very little liquid remains. Remove from the heat and fold in the goat cheese.

3. Toast the bread and place each slice on a plate. Spread the toast with the remaining 2 teaspoons (10 mL) ghee and top with the scrambled eggs. Finish with a sprinkle of pepper.

◆ **Gluten-Free:** Use gluten-free bread instead of sourdough bread.

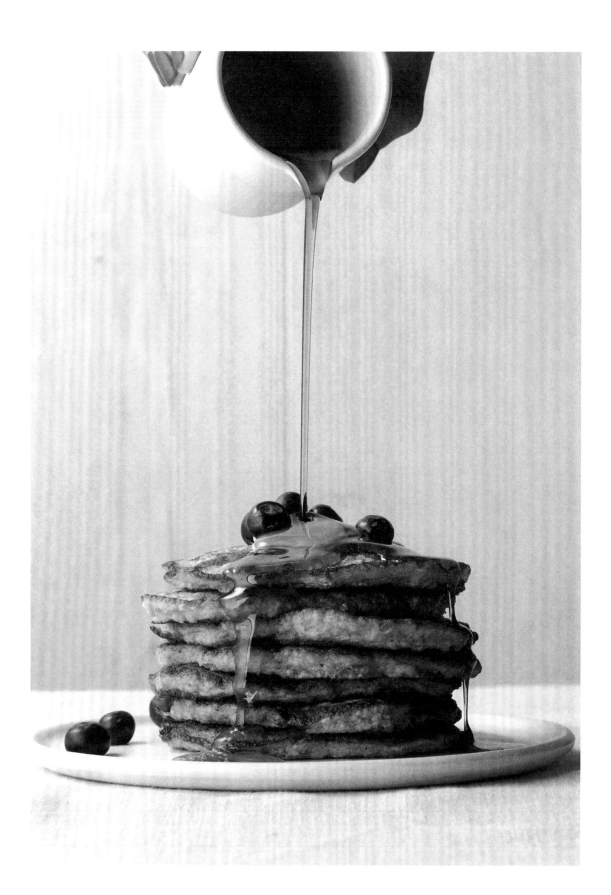

Easy Banana Oat Pancakes

These pancakes are gluten-free, dairy-free, and full of healthy fats, protein, and fibre. They don't bubble up as much as regular pancakes, so you'll have to check the bottom for doneness. They are quite delicate, so it is best to use a nonstick pan to make it easy to flip them. I love topping them with maple syrup, ghee, and blueberries, but feel free to get creative with the toppings and let your imagination run wild!

½ cup (125 mL) gluten-free rolled oats

3 pasture-raised or organic eggs

2 very ripe bananas

1 teaspoon (5 mL) baking powder

Pinch of sea salt

Ghee, Plain Jane Ghee (page 271), or virgin coconut oil, for frying

To Serve

Ghee or Plain Jane Ghee (page 271), at room temperature

Pure maple syrup

Fresh blueberries

1. In a food processor, process the oats until ground to a powder-like consistency, 45 to 60 seconds.

2. Add the eggs, bananas, baking powder, and salt. Blend until smooth.

3. Brush a large nonstick pan lightly with ghee and heat over medium heat. When the pan is hot, pour in ⅓ cup (75 mL) of the batter per pancake, cooking 2 to 3 pancakes at a time. Cook for 1 to 2 minutes per side, flipping when bubbles form around the edges. Repeat with the remaining batter, brushing the pan lightly with ghee between each batch of pancakes.

4. To serve, top the pancakes with ghee, maple syrup, and blueberries or your favourite toppings.

Crispy Almond Flour Waffles with Coconut Whipped Cream

These are the best grain-free waffles you will ever have! They are crispy on the outside, fluffy on the inside, and very satisfying in every way. They do require a few steps and a fair amount of dishes, so I suggest reserving them for leisurely weekend breakfasts. You can also make a batch ahead of time and keep them in the freezer for quick weekday breakfasts. All you have to do is pop them in the toaster and add your favourite toppings!

3 cups (750 mL) super-fine blanched almond flour

½ cup (125 mL) tapioca starch

⅓ cup (75 mL) coconut sugar

1 teaspoon (5 mL) baking soda

½ teaspoon (2 mL) sea salt

1 cup (250 mL) unsweetened almond milk

4 pasture-raised or organic eggs, separated

¼ cup (60 mL) ghee or Plain Jane Ghee (page 271), melted, more for the waffle iron

1 teaspoon (5 mL) apple cider vinegar

1 teaspoon (5 mL) pure vanilla extract or ½ teaspoon (2 mL) pure vanilla powder

To Serve

Coconut Whipped Cream (page 274)

Pure maple syrup

Fresh berries

1. Preheat the oven to 200°F (100°C).
2. In a large bowl, whisk together the almond flour, tapioca starch, coconut sugar, baking soda, and salt.
3. In a medium bowl, whisk together the almond milk, egg yolks, ghee, apple cider vinegar, and vanilla. Add the egg mixture to the almond flour mixture and whisk to combine.
4. In another medium bowl, add the egg whites. Using electric beaters, beat the egg whites until soft peaks form. Using a spatula, scoop the beaten egg whites into the waffle batter and gently fold in.
5. Preheat the waffle iron on a medium-high setting. Lightly brush the waffle iron with ghee.
6. When the ready light comes on, pour about ⅔ cup (150 mL) batter into the centre of the waffle iron. Cook until crispy and golden brown, 2 to 3 minutes.
7. Using tongs, remove the waffle and place it directly on a rack in the oven to keep warm. Repeat with the remaining batter, lightly brushing the waffle iron with ghee before cooking each waffle.
8. To serve, top the waffles with Coconut Whipped Cream, a drizzle of maple syrup, and fresh berries.

◆ **Paleo-Friendly:** Use pure vanilla powder instead of pure vanilla extract.

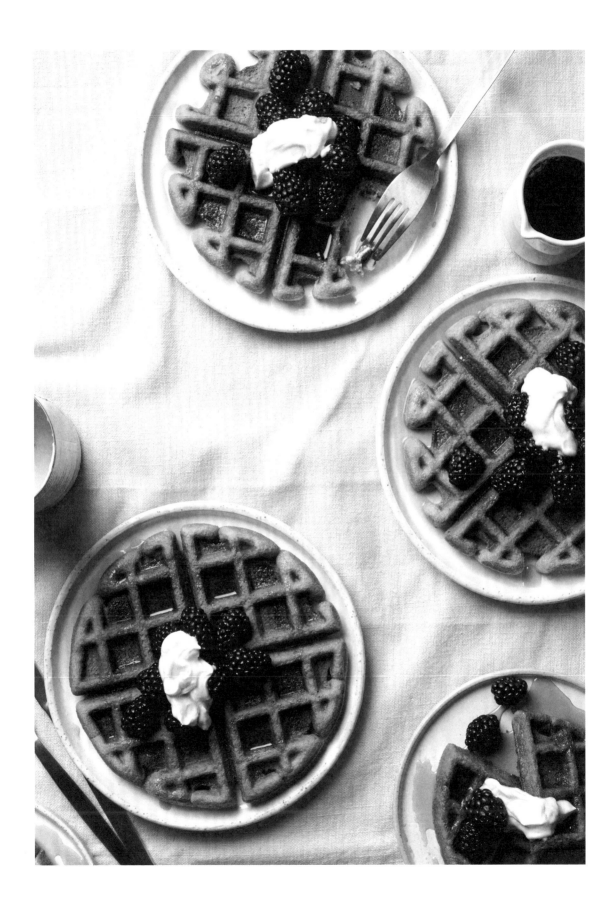

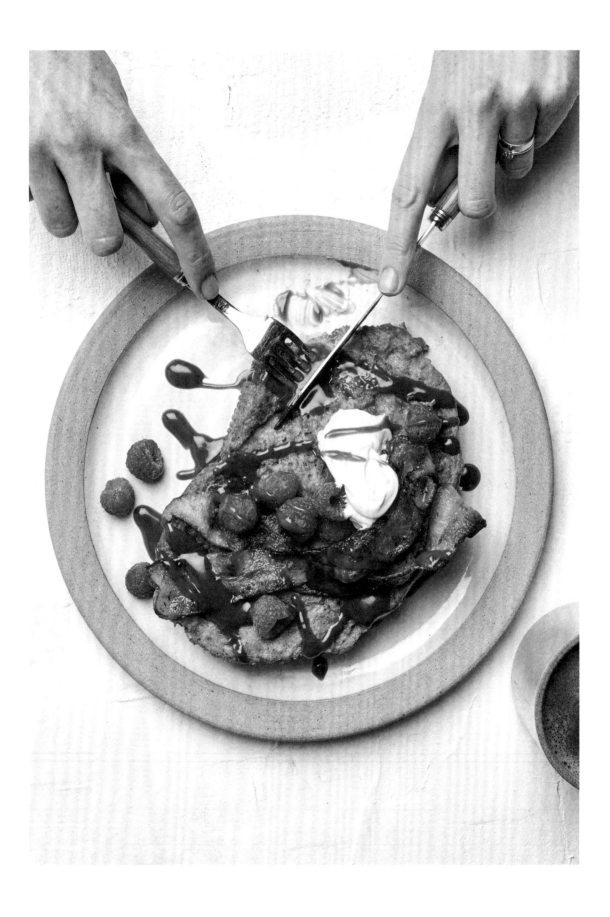

Sourdough French Toast with Bacon

On one Christmas morning I will never forget, my mother strayed from her usual bacon and egg breakfast spread. Instead, she made French toast, complete with an array of toppings to choose from and crispy bacon on the side. It was pure heaven. This recipe uses sourdough bread for a light, fluffy texture. The French toast is served with coconut milk dulce de leche and coconut whipped cream, making it appropriate for those who can't have dairy. This recipe is excellent for larger groups and for when you want something that feels like a special treat.

Sourdough French Toast

8 pasture-raised or organic eggs

1 can (14 ounces/398 mL) full-fat coconut milk, divided

1 teaspoon (5 mL) cinnamon

¼ teaspoon (1 mL) pure vanilla extract

8 slices of bread from a sourdough boule, cut ½-inch (1 cm) thick

Ghee or Plain Jane Ghee (page 271), for frying

Dulce de Coco

½ cup (125 mL) coconut sugar

½ teaspoon (2 mL) sea salt

1 tablespoon (15 mL) ghee or Plain Jane Ghee (page 271), at room temperature

½ teaspoon (2 mL) pure vanilla extract

To Serve

Coconut Whipped Cream (page 274)

Fresh berries

1 pound (450 g) Perfect Oven Bacon (page 270)

1. Position a rack in the middle of the oven. Preheat the oven to 200°F (100°C).

2. **Make the Sourdough French Toast** In a large bowl, whisk the eggs. Add 2 tablespoons (30 mL) coconut milk, along with the cinnamon and vanilla. Whisk to combine. Pour the mixture into a 12½- × 8½-inch (3.5 L) baking dish. Soak the bread slices in the mixture for 2 minutes per side.

3. In a large skillet over medium-high heat, heat 1 tablespoon (15 mL) ghee. Lay 2 slices of bread in the pan. Cook until golden brown, 3 to 4 minutes per side.

4. Using tongs, remove the French toast from the pan and place it directly on the rack in the oven to keep warm. Cook the remaining French toast, 2 slices at a time, adding a bit more ghee to the pan before frying each batch. Wipe the pan clean.

5. **Make the Dulce de Coco** In the same skillet over medium-high heat, add the remaining coconut milk. Bring to a simmer, then reduce the heat to medium. Stir in the coconut sugar and salt and simmer, stirring constantly, until the mixture thickens to a sticky, caramel-like consistency, 5 to 10 minutes. Remove from the heat and stir in the ghee and vanilla.

6. To serve, top the French toast with a dollop of Coconut Whipped Cream, a drizzle of Dulce de Coco, and fresh berries. Serve with Perfect Oven Bacon.

◆ **Gluten-Free:** Use gluten-free bread instead of sourdough bread.
Vegetarian: Skip the Perfect Oven Bacon.

Grainless Ghee-nola

This buttery granola is full of large, crunchy clusters. I always have a jar on hand for snacking or to add some crunch to breakfast bowls. This granola is packed with healthy omega-3 fatty acids from nuts, seeds, and a whole egg. It is not too sweet and will help keep you energized with good fats throughout the day.

2 cups (500 mL) raw walnuts

2 cups (500 mL) raw whole almonds

1 cup (250 mL) raw pumpkin seeds

1 cup (250 mL) unsweetened shredded coconut

½ cup (125 mL) raw sesame seeds

½ cup (125 mL) raw sunflower seeds

¼ cup (60 mL) coconut sugar

2 tablespoons (30 mL) chia seeds

1 teaspoon (5 mL) cinnamon

½ teaspoon (2 mL) sea salt

6 tablespoons (90 mL) ghee or Plain Jane Ghee (page 271), melted

½ cup (125 mL) pure maple syrup

1 pasture-raised or organic egg

1. Preheat the oven to 300°F (150°C). Line a baking sheet with parchment paper.

2. In a large bowl, combine the walnuts, almonds, pumpkin seeds, shredded coconut, sesame seeds, sunflower seeds, coconut sugar, chia seeds, cinnamon, and salt.

3. In a small bowl, mix together the ghee and maple syrup. Add the ghee mixture to the nut mixture and stir to combine.

4. In the same small bowl (no need to wipe it clean), whisk the egg until frothy and pale yellow. Add the whisked egg to the granola mixture and stir to combine.

5. Spread the granola evenly on the prepared baking sheet and bake until golden brown, 35 to 40 minutes, stirring once halfway through the baking time. Oven temperatures vary, so be sure to keep a close eye on the granola so it does not burn. Remove from the oven and let cool for 10 minutes without stirring. This will help form large clusters. Store in an air-tight container in the fridge for up to 1 month.

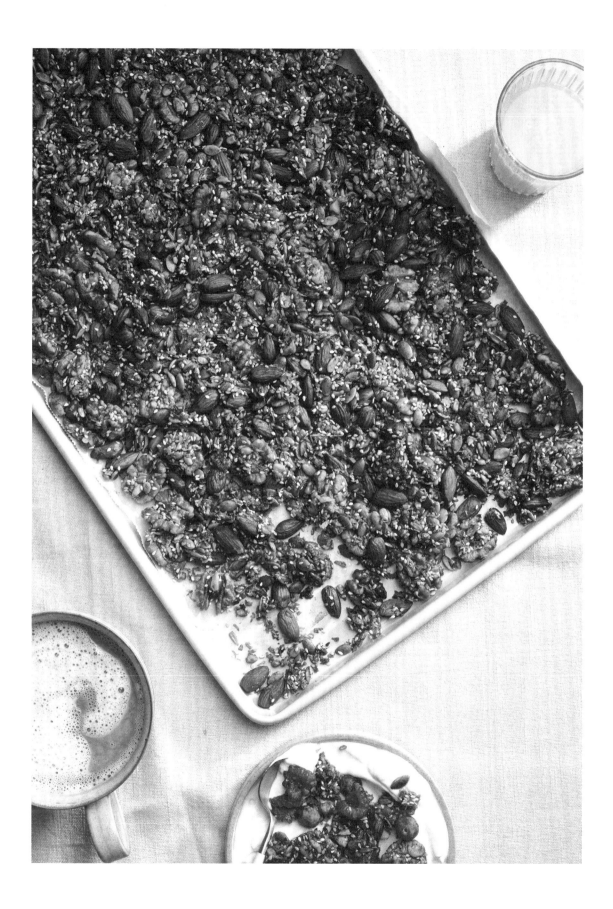

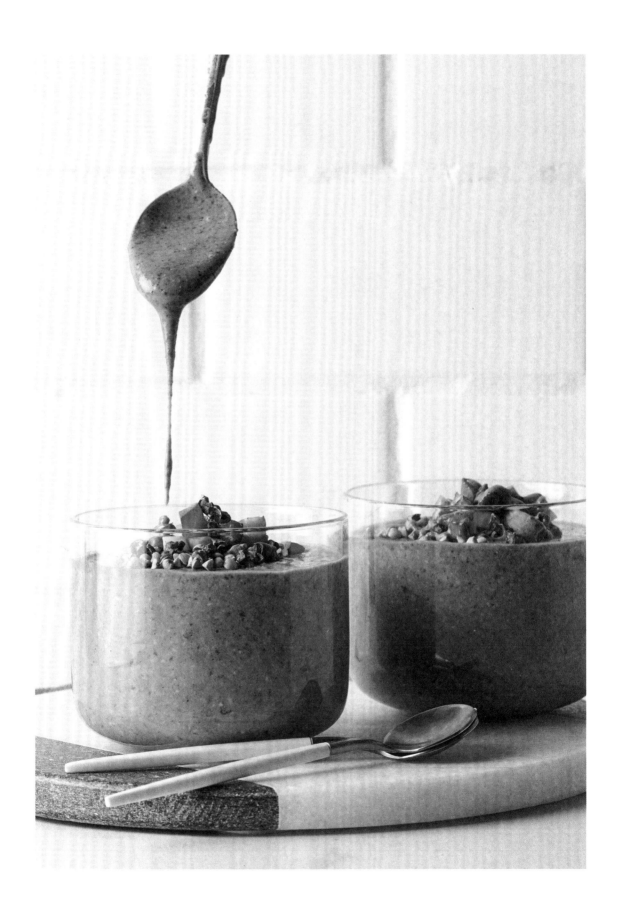

Dairy-Free ◆ Gluten-Free ◆ Vegan ◆ *Serves 2*

Buckwheat Chia Pudding with Almond Butter Drizzle

Although chia puddings are as plentiful as the day is long, if you haven't tried adding toasted buckwheat to a chia pudding before, you are in for a real treat. Buckwheat adds a nutty, earthy flavour and skin-loving antioxidants that help you glow from the inside out. Despite its misleading name, buckwheat is a seed, not a grain, which makes it suitable for those on gluten-free diets. The cacao powder adds a subtle chocolate flavour, but you can just as easily leave it out if you prefer.

½ cup (125 mL) + 1 tablespoon (15 mL) raw buckwheat groats

1½ cups (375 mL) unsweetened almond milk

1 banana

1 tablespoon (15 mL) chia seeds

1 tablespoon (15 mL) flax seeds

1 tablespoon (15 mL) cacao powder (optional)

1 tablespoon (15 mL) pure maple syrup

Pinch of sea salt

To Serve

Raw cacao nibs

Fresh strawberries, chopped

Natural almond butter or Homemade Almond Butter (page 275), to drizzle

1. Heat a dry, large skillet over medium-high heat. Add the buckwheat groats in a single layer. Toast, tossing occasionally, until fragrant and lightly browned, 5 to 6 minutes.

2. Transfer the toasted buckwheat to a high-speed blender or food processor, reserving 1 tablespoon (15 mL) to top the pudding. Add the almond milk, banana, chia seeds, flax seeds, cacao powder (if using), maple syrup, and salt. Blend until smooth, 15 to 20 seconds.

3. Pour the mixture into 2 small serving dishes. Cover and refrigerate overnight (the mixture will thicken as it sets). In the morning, serve topped with the reserved toasted buckwheat, cacao nibs, and strawberries. Drizzle with almond butter.

Buttered Steel-Cut Oatmeal with Caramelized Banana

Steel-cut oats are a great source of fibre and nutrients. Adding ghee to the oats after cooking makes them creamy and buttery. The almond butter and Grainless Ghee-nola (page 52) toppings provide a fullness-inducing combination of fibre, protein, and fats that helps keep you satisfied for hours. Most importantly, the caramelized bananas make this humble bowl of oats taste just like banana bread. Soaking the steel-cut oats ahead of time reduces the cooking time and makes them easier to digest.

Oatmeal

1 cup (250 mL) gluten-free steel-cut oats

Pinch of sea salt

1 tablespoon + 1½ teaspoons (22 mL) ghee, Plain Jane Ghee (page 271), or organic unsalted butter, at room temperature

¾ teaspoon (4 mL) cinnamon

¼ teaspoon (1 mL) pure vanilla extract

Caramelized Bananas

1 teaspoon (5 mL) ghee, Plain Jane Ghee (page 271), or virgin coconut oil

2 bananas, sliced in half lengthwise

To Serve

Plain full-fat yogurt or plain coconut yogurt

Natural almond butter or Homemade Almond Butter (page 275), to drizzle

Pure maple syrup

Grainless Ghee-nola (page 52) or nuts and seeds

1. Place the oats in a medium bowl and cover them with filtered water. Cover the bowl with a kitchen towel and soak overnight at room temperature. Using a fine mesh strainer, drain and rinse the oats thoroughly.

2. **Cook the Oatmeal** In a medium saucepan, add the soaked oats, 1½ cups (375 mL) water, and salt. Cover and bring to a boil over high heat. Reduce the heat to medium-low and simmer, covered, stirring occasionally, until the water is absorbed and the oats are soft, 10 to 12 minutes. Stir in the ghee, cinnamon, and vanilla.

3. **Caramelize the Bananas** In a medium nonstick pan over medium heat, heat the ghee. Add the banana slices, cut side down, and cook, undisturbed, until golden brown on the bottom, 5 to 7 minutes. Flip and cook for 1 to 2 minutes on the other side.

4. To serve, divide the oatmeal between 2 bowls. Top each bowl with caramelized bananas and a dollop of yogurt. Drizzle with almond butter and maple syrup. Finish with a sprinkle of Grainless Ghee-nola for crunch.

◆ **Dairy-Free:** Use coconut yogurt instead of dairy yogurt. **Nut-Free:** Skip the almond butter and Grainless Ghee-nola. **Vegan:** Use coconut yogurt instead of dairy yogurt. Use virgin coconut oil instead of ghee. Skip the Grainless Ghee-nola.

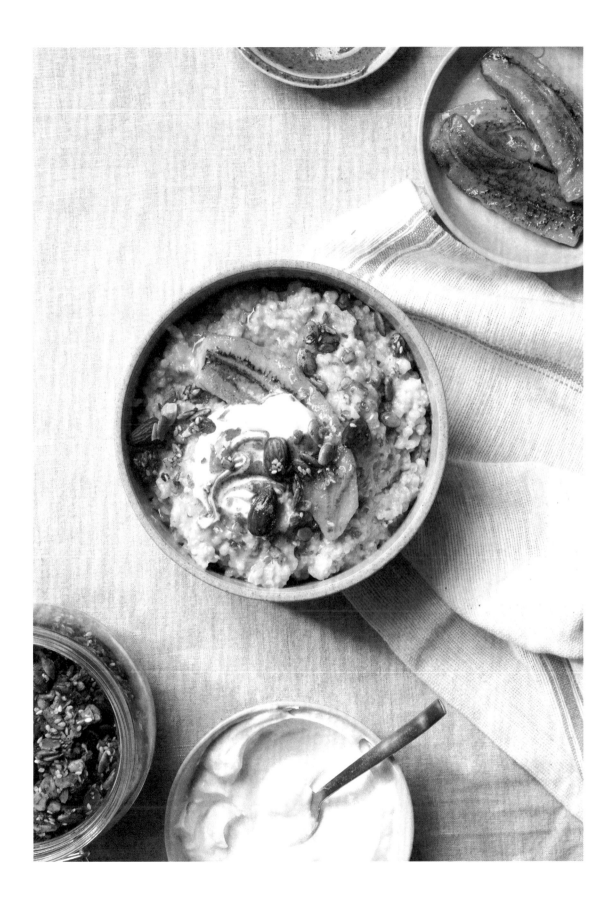

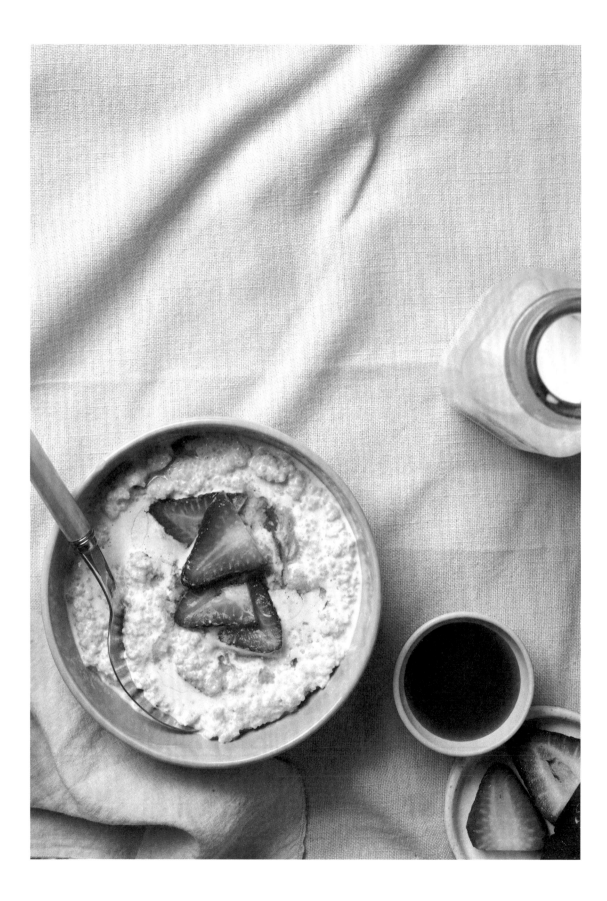

Creamy Millet Porridge

This is an incredibly tasty porridge made with millet—one of my favourite grains. Toasting the millet adds a nutty flavour and helps it keep its shape during cooking—this step is optional. The recipe gets its creaminess from whole goat's milk (but you can substitute whole cow's milk or macadamia milk if you prefer). As the milk reduces on the stove, it encapsulates each grain of millet. This gruel will sustain you for hours, and the texture is divine!

½ cup (125 mL) millet

2 cups (500 mL) whole goat's milk, more to serve

⅛ teaspoon (0.5 mL) ground cardamom

Pinch of sea salt

To Serve

Fresh berries

Pure maple syrup

1. Heat a dry, large skillet over medium-high heat. Add the millet in a single layer. Toast, tossing occasionally, until fragrant and lightly browned, 5 to 6 minutes.

2. In a medium saucepan, add the millet, goat's milk, cardamom, and salt and bring to a boil over high heat. Reduce the heat to medium-low and cook, uncovered, stirring often, until all of the milk is absorbed and the mixture is thick and creamy, 12 to 15 minutes.

3. To serve, divide the porridge between 2 bowls. Top with fresh berries, a drizzle of maple syrup, and another splash of goat's milk for good measure.

◆ **Dairy-Free and Vegan:** Use macadamia milk (see page 273) instead of goat's milk.

Crispy Sweet Potato Egg Nests

These egg nests are a healthy and delicious way to start the day that reminds me of my favourite childhood breakfast, toad-in-the-hole. In this version, the ghee adds a rich, buttery flavour and gives the sweet potato nest delightfully crispy edges. A spiralizer is required to make noodle shapes from the sweet potato. Reserve the leftover egg yolk to make Healthyish Carbonara (page 132).

1 small sweet potato, peeled

¼ cup (60 mL) ghee or Plain Jane Ghee (page 271), divided

1 teaspoon (5 mL) garlic powder

¼ teaspoon (1 mL) sea salt

Pinch of black pepper

2 pasture-raised or organic eggs

1 pasture-raised or organic egg white

To Serve

Pinch of red chili flakes

1 avocado, peeled, pitted, and sliced

1 tomato, sliced

Hot sauce (optional)

1. Using a spiralizer fitted with the smallest attachment, spiralize the sweet potato. Using kitchen scissors, cut the pieces into spaghetti lengths so that they are easier to work with.

2. In a large skillet over medium-high heat, melt 2 tablespoons (30 mL) of the ghee. Add the sweet potato noodles and sprinkle them with the garlic powder, salt, and pepper. Sauté, stirring often, until softened, 8 to 10 minutes.

3. Reduce the heat to medium-low. Arrange the sweet potato noodles in 2 circular nest shapes in the pan. Using a spatula or a spoon, create a well in the centre of each nest, large enough to hold an egg yolk comfortably.

4. Crack 1 egg into each well. Cook, uncovered, until the whites of the eggs are nearly set, 8 to 10 minutes. Sprinkle a bit more salt and pepper on the egg yolks.

5. While the eggs are cooking, spoon half of the egg white over each of the nests, to help the sweet potato stick together.

6. Add the remaining 2 tablespoons (30 mL) ghee to the edge of the pan. Increase the heat to high. When the ghee is hot, carefully tilt the pan and spoon the ghee over the egg whites, avoiding the yolks. The whites will bubble and become fully set, while the yolks will stay runny.

7. To serve, place each nest on a plate and sprinkle with chili flakes. Serve with sliced avocado, sliced tomatoes, and hot sauce, if using.

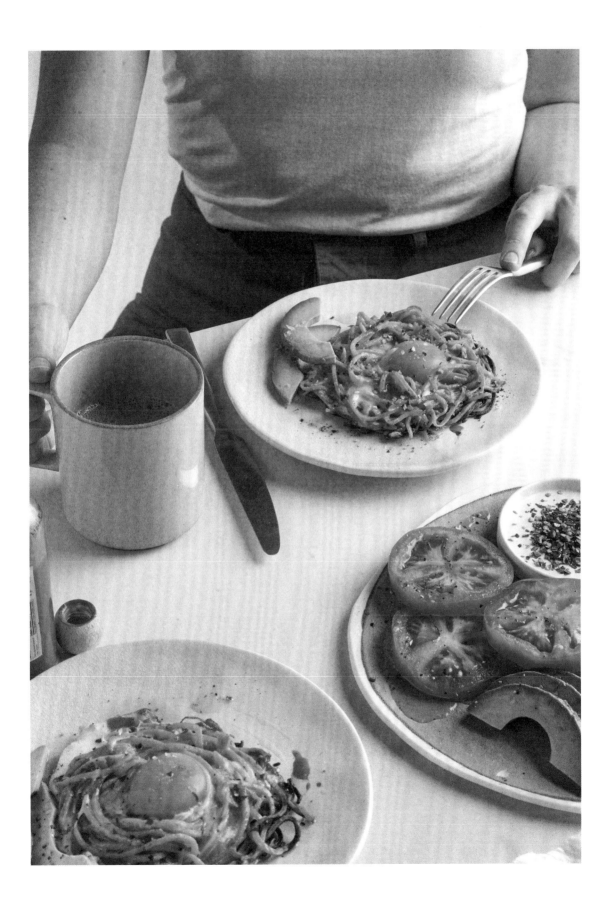

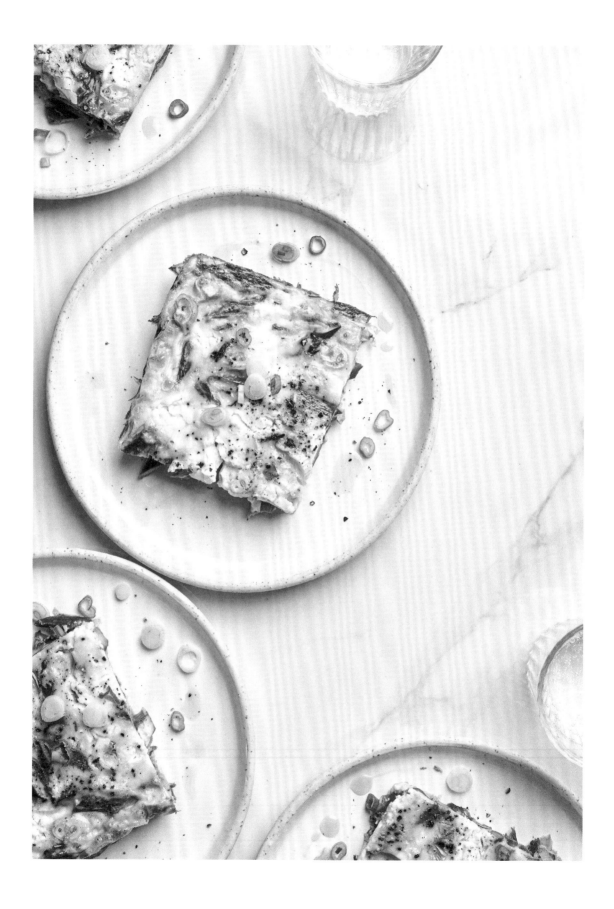

Spring Asparagus and Goat Cheese Frittata

This simple spring frittata is a great way to use the abundance of asparagus when it is in season. It is full of healthy fats and protein and is low in carbohydrates, which means it will help keep your blood sugar and energy levels stable throughout the day. Look for the thinnest asparagus spears you can find, as they are more tender and cook quicker. This frittata is delicious served hot or cold, so you can make it ahead and have it for grab-and-go breakfasts during the week. Feel free to substitute other vegetables, such as spinach, mushrooms, or peppers.

8 pasture-raised or organic eggs

½ cup (125 mL) full-fat canned coconut milk

Sea salt and black pepper, to taste

1 tablespoon (15 mL) ghee, Plain Jane Ghee (page 271), or avocado oil, more for the pan

1 bunch of thin asparagus, ends trimmed and sliced into ½-inch (1 cm) pieces

⅔ cup (150 mL) crumbled goat cheese

1 bunch of green onions (white and light green parts only), thinly sliced

Hot sauce, to serve (optional)

1. Position a rack in the middle of the oven. Preheat the oven to 350°F (180°C). Grease a glass 8-inch (2 L) square baking dish with ghee.

2. In a large bowl, whisk the eggs until frothy and pale yellow. Whisk in the coconut milk, salt, and pepper.

3. In a large cast-iron skillet over medium-high heat, heat the ghee. Add the asparagus and sauté, stirring occasionally, until tender, 4 to 6 minutes. Add the cooked asparagus, goat cheese, and green onion to the egg mixture and stir to combine. Transfer to the prepared baking dish. Bake until the frittata puffs up and turns golden brown, 25 to 30 minutes.

4. Cut into 4 squares and serve hot or cold with hot sauce, if using. Store leftover frittata in an airtight container in the fridge for up to 4 days.

Dairy-Free ◆ Gluten-Free Option ◆ Grain-Free Option ◆ Nut-Free ◆ Keto-Friendly Option ◆
Paleo-Friendly Option ◆ *Serves 2 to 4*

Eggs Florentine with Smoked Salmon and Ghee Hollandaise

This recipe is a powerhouse of nutrition that will give you loads of energy. I would eat this every day if I could! The hollandaise is dense and buttery, and the pasture-raised eggs and smoked salmon provide those fantastic omega-3 fatty acids. You can poach the eggs after making the ghee hollandaise. The sprouted whole-grain English muffins are delicious (I use the Ezekiel brand), but if you would rather eat fewer carbs, feel free to leave them out.

Sautéed Spinach

2 tablespoons (30 mL) avocado oil

4 cups (1 L) tightly packed baby spinach

Pinch of sea salt

Ghee Hollandaise

2 pasture-raised or organic egg yolks

1 tablespoon + 1½ teaspoons (22 mL) fresh lemon juice

½ teaspoon (2 mL) sea salt

½ cup (125 mL) melted ghee or Plain Jane Ghee (page 271)

To Serve

2 sprouted whole-grain English muffins, cut in half (optional)

2 teaspoons (10 mL) ghee or Plain Jane Ghee (page 271), at room temperature

2½ ounces (70 g) smoked sockeye salmon

4 Poached Eggs (page 268)

1. **Make the Sautéed Spinach** In a large skillet over medium-high heat, heat the avocado oil. Add the spinach and salt. Sauté, stirring occasionally, until the spinach is just wilted, 1 to 2 minutes. Remove from the heat and cover to keep warm.

2. **Make the Ghee Hollandaise** In a high-speed blender, combine the egg yolks, lemon juice, and salt. Reduce the speed to low and slowly pour in the melted ghee. Process until the sauce emulsifies and becomes thick and creamy, 1 to 2 minutes.

3. To serve, toast the English muffins (if using) and spread all 4 halves with ghee. Divide the Sautéed Spinach between the 4 halves. Top each with smoked salmon and a poached egg. Pour the Ghee Hollandaise over top. Serve immediately.

◆ **Gluten-Free:** Use gluten-free English muffins instead of sprouted whole-grain muffins.

Grain-Free, Keto-Friendly, and Paleo-Friendly: Skip the toasted English muffins.

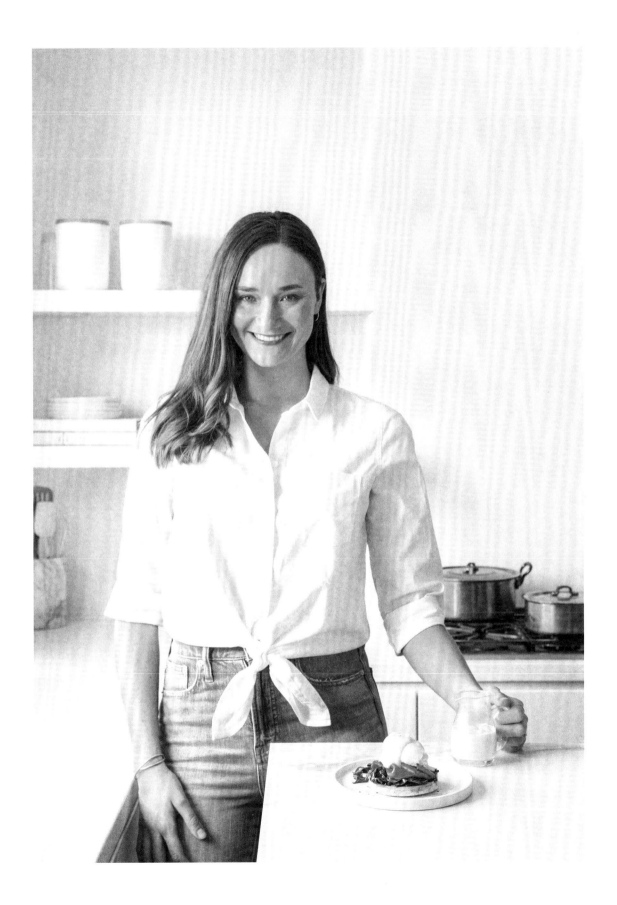

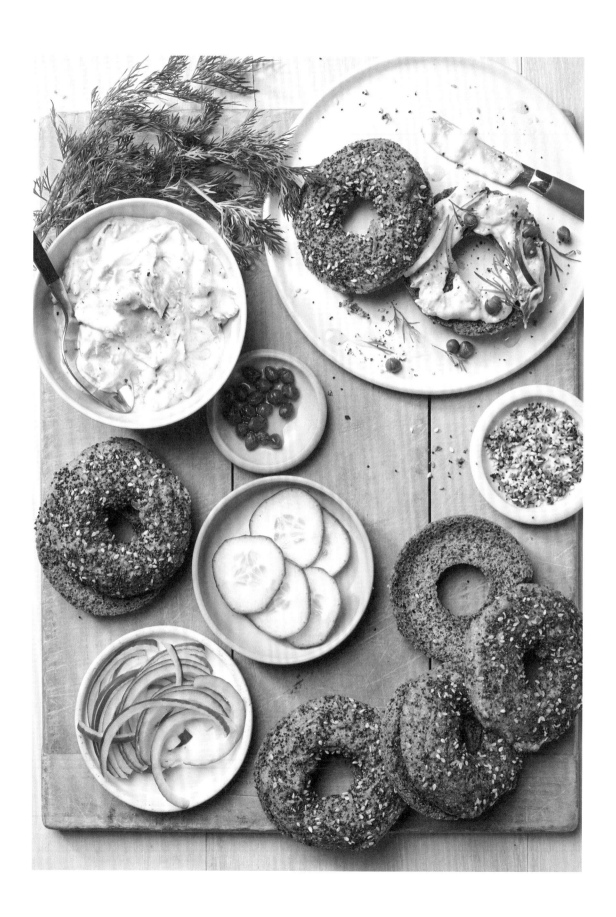

Grain-Free Everything Bagels with Smoked Trout Spread

This delicious bagel recipe was developed by Jessica Stupak, a holistic nutritionist I work with. These bagels are smaller than regular ones, but since they are made from almond flour, they are very filling and satisfying. My favourite way to serve them is smeared with my fresh, lemony smoked trout spread for breakfast. The spread is made simply by combining omega-3-rich smoked trout with my Lemon Aioli (page 277). Just be sure to source the fish from a fishmonger you trust, because quality makes a huge difference here.

Grain-Free Everything Bagels

1 cup (250 mL) super-fine blanched almond flour

⅓ cup (75 mL) ground flaxseed

1 teaspoon (5 mL) baking soda

¼ teaspoon (1 mL) sea salt

3 pasture-raised or organic eggs

2 tablespoons (30 mL) avocado oil, more for the pan

2 teaspoons (10 mL) apple cider vinegar

1½ teaspoons (7 mL) sesame seeds

1 teaspoon (5 mL) poppy seeds

1 teaspoon (5 mL) dried garlic flakes

1 teaspoon (5 mL) dried onion flakes

Smoked Trout Spread

6 ounces (170 g) sugar-free smoked trout, flaked into chunks

½ cup (125 mL) Lemon Aioli (page 277)

¼ teaspoon (1 mL) sweet paprika

Pinch of black pepper

To Serve

Sliced cucumber

Sliced red onion

Chopped fresh dill

Capers, drained

1. Preheat the oven to 350°F (180°C). Lightly grease a 6-cavity doughnut pan with avocado oil.
2. **Make the Grain-Free Everything Bagels** In a large bowl, combine the almond flour, flaxseed, baking soda, and salt.
3. In a small bowl, whisk together the eggs, avocado oil, and apple cider vinegar.
4. Add the egg mixture to the flour mixture and stir to combine. Carefully spoon the batter into the doughnut pan, filling each cavity about three-quarters full. Smooth out the top of the batter.
5. In a small bowl, combine the sesame seeds, poppy seeds, garlic flakes, and onion flakes. Sprinkle the mixture over the bagel batter. Bake until the bagels are golden brown on the outside, 25 to 30 minutes. Place the pan on a rack and let cool in the pan for 10 to 15 minutes before removing the bagels from the pan. Cool completely, 15 to 20 minutes.
6. **Make the Smoked Trout Spread** In a small bowl, mix together the smoked trout, Lemon Aioli, paprika, and pepper.
7. To serve, slice the bagels in half and toast them. Spread a generous layer of Smoked Trout Spread on each bagel. Top with sliced cucumber and red onion, dill, and capers. Store leftover bagels in an airtight container in the freezer for up to 1 month.

Warming Sweet Potato Breakfast Bowl with Almond Butter Drizzle

This cozy breakfast bowl is inspired by the ancient system of Ayurveda, which teaches that during the colder winter months it is best to eat foods that are warming, grounding, and full of healthy fats to balance the body. The sweet potato, ghee, and chai spice combo deliver precisely that! I suggest roasting the sweet potato ahead of time, so that all you have to do is blend everything together. The Grainless Ghee-nola (page 52) and coconut flakes add a delightful, fat-filled crunch.

1 large sweet potato

1 cup (250 mL) unsweetened almond milk

1 banana

2 teaspoons (10 mL) ghee or Plain Jane Ghee (page 271), at room temperature

½ teaspoon (2 mL) cinnamon

¼ teaspoon (1 mL) ground ginger

¼ teaspoon (1 mL) nutmeg

Pinch of ground cloves

Pinch of sea salt

To Serve

Grainless Ghee-nola (page 52) or store-bought granola

Unsweetened coconut flakes

Natural almond butter or Homemade Almond Butter (page 275), to drizzle

1. Preheat the oven to 375°F (190°C). Line a baking sheet with parchment paper.

2. Slice the sweet potato in half lengthwise. Place the potato halves, cut side down, on the prepared baking sheet. Using the tip of a knife, make prick marks all over the skin. Roast until fork-tender, 25 to 30 minutes. Using a spoon, scoop out the flesh of the sweet potato and transfer it to a high-speed blender.

3. In a small saucepan over medium-high heat, warm the almond milk for 1 to 2 minutes, then pour it into the blender. Add the banana, ghee, cinnamon, ginger, nutmeg, cloves, and salt. Blend on high speed until smooth, 15 to 20 seconds.

4. To serve, divide the sweet potato purée between 2 bowls. Sprinkle with Grainless Ghee-nola and coconut flakes. Drizzle almond butter over top.

◆ **Vegan:** Use virgin coconut oil instead of ghee. Skip the Grainless Ghee-nola.

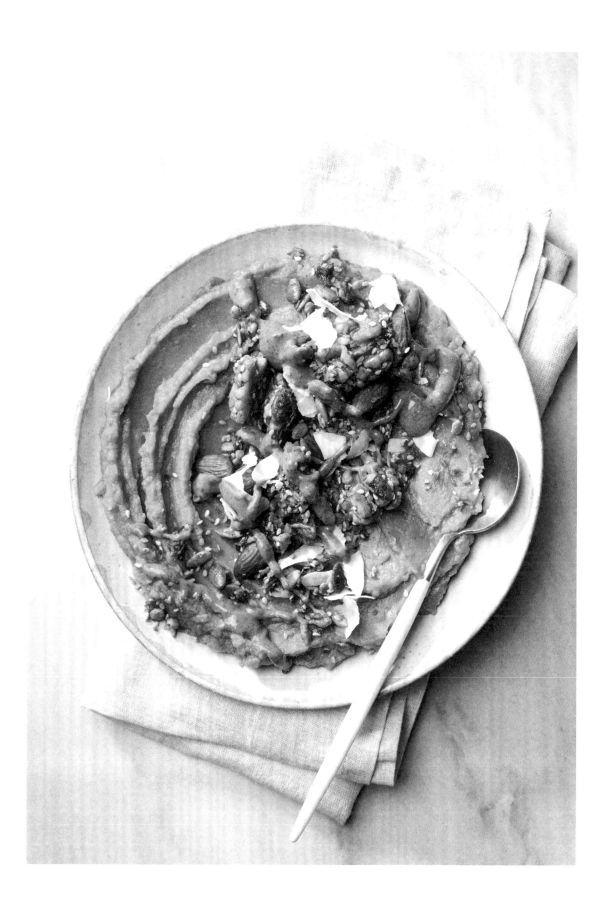

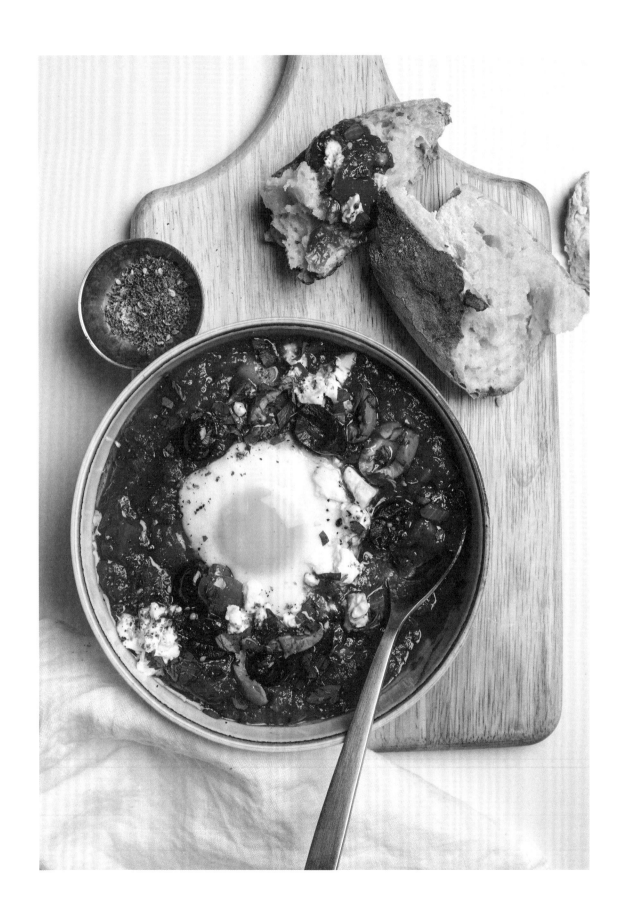

◆ Shakshuka with Olives, Feta, and Za'atar

Some of my favourite memories (such as my first date with my husband) were made over this Middle Eastern dish. This shakshuka is inexpensive and straightforward and feeds a crowd—it can be served for a nice brunch with friends or as an easy weeknight dinner. Harissa paste is sold at specialty food shops, but feel free to leave it out or substitute another chili-based hot sauce if you cannot find it. Extra-virgin olive oil adds the appropriate flavour profile, and the delicious, fat-fuelled toppings take this classic dish to a whole new level!

3 tablespoons (45 mL) extra-virgin olive oil, more to serve

1 medium yellow onion, diced

1 red bell pepper, seeded and diced

2 cloves garlic, minced

1 tablespoon (15 mL) ground cumin

1 tablespoon (15 mL) smoked paprika

1 tablespoon (15 mL) mild harissa paste or other chili-based hot sauce (optional)

1 can (28 ounces/796 mL) crushed tomatoes

1 teaspoon (5 mL) lemon zest

1 teaspoon (5 mL) sea salt

¼ teaspoon (1 mL) black pepper

6 pasture-raised or organic eggs

To Serve

¼ cup (60 mL) pitted black or green olives, chopped

1 ounce (28 g) crumbled sheep's or goat's milk feta cheese

1 teaspoon (5 mL) za'atar

¼ cup (60 mL) loosely packed chopped fresh flat-leaf parsley

Crusty whole-grain sourdough bread (optional)

1. In a 10-inch (25 cm) cast-iron skillet over medium heat, heat the olive oil. Add the onion and bell pepper. Cook, stirring occasionally, until softened, 10 to 12 minutes.

2. Add the garlic, cumin, paprika, and harissa paste, if using. Stir to combine. Cook for 1 minute until fragrant.

3. Stir in the tomatoes, lemon zest, salt, and pepper. Bring the sauce to a simmer over medium heat. Simmer, stirring occasionally, until slightly thickened, 3 to 5 minutes. Reduce the heat to low.

4. Using a spoon, create a well in the sauce near the edge of the pan. Crack an egg into the well. Create 4 more wells along the edge of the pan, cracking an egg into each one. Lastly, create a well in the centre of the pan and crack the remaining egg into it. Cover the skillet with an inverted 10-inch (25 cm) frying pan or a large plate. Cook over low heat until the egg whites are set and the yolks are still soft and runny, 18 to 20 minutes. Remove from the heat.

5. Scatter the shakshuka with the olives, crumbled feta, and za'atar. Drizzle with olive oil and top with the parsley.

6. To serve, carefully scoop out the eggs with the sauce and place in serving bowls. Serve with warm sourdough bread, if desired.

◆ **Gluten-Free, Grain-Free, Keto-Friendly, and Paleo-Friendly:** Skip the sourdough bread.

◆ Power Greens Breakfast

This is my go-to breakfast when I need a boost of energy to get me through a busy day. Egg yolks are a great source of good fats. Plus, when you pair eggs with leafy greens, you actually get more of the nutrients from the greens. They are a power combo, hence the name of this recipe. To save time on preparation, you can buy pre-washed chopped kale and poach the eggs while you sauté the kale. Serving the dish with avocado adds extra good fats, and a squeeze of lime juice gives it some brightness.

3 tablespoons (45 mL) ghee, Plain Jane Ghee (page 271), or avocado oil

4 cloves garlic, thinly sliced

6 cups (1.5 L) packed chopped curly green kale, stems and ribs removed

¼ teaspoon (1 mL) ground cumin

¼ teaspoon (1 mL) sweet paprika

¼ teaspoon (1 mL) sea salt

2 Poached Eggs (page 268)

Pinch of red chili flakes

To Serve

Sliced avocado

Fresh lime wedges

1. In a large skillet over medium-high heat, heat the ghee. Add the sliced garlic and cook until it just starts to brown, about 1 minute.

2. Add the chopped kale, cumin, paprika, and salt. Using tongs, toss to coat. Sauté, tossing frequently, until the kale is wilted and tender, 4 to 5 minutes.

3. To serve, divide the greens between 2 plates. Top with a poached egg and a sprinkle of chili flakes. Serve with sliced avocado and lime wedges.

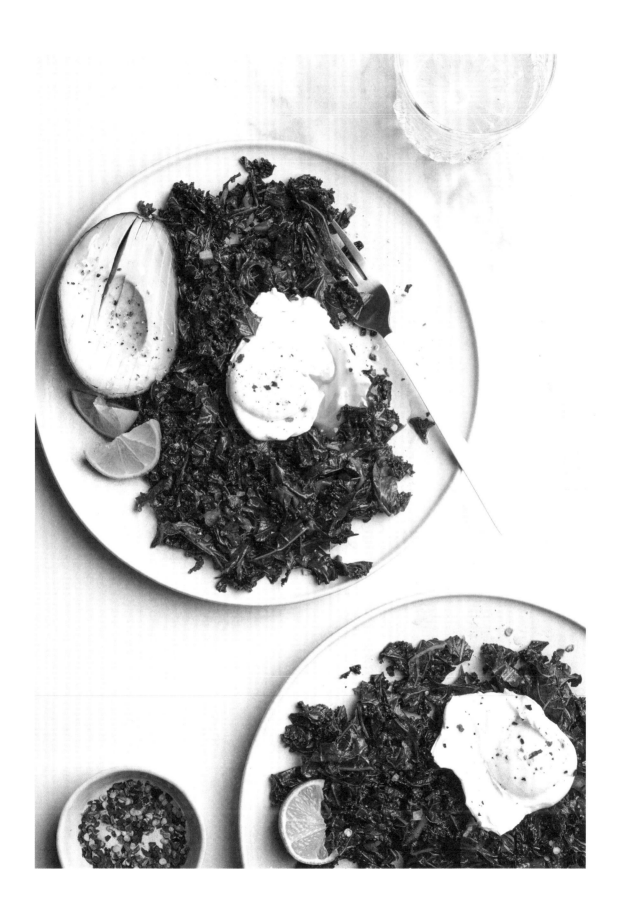

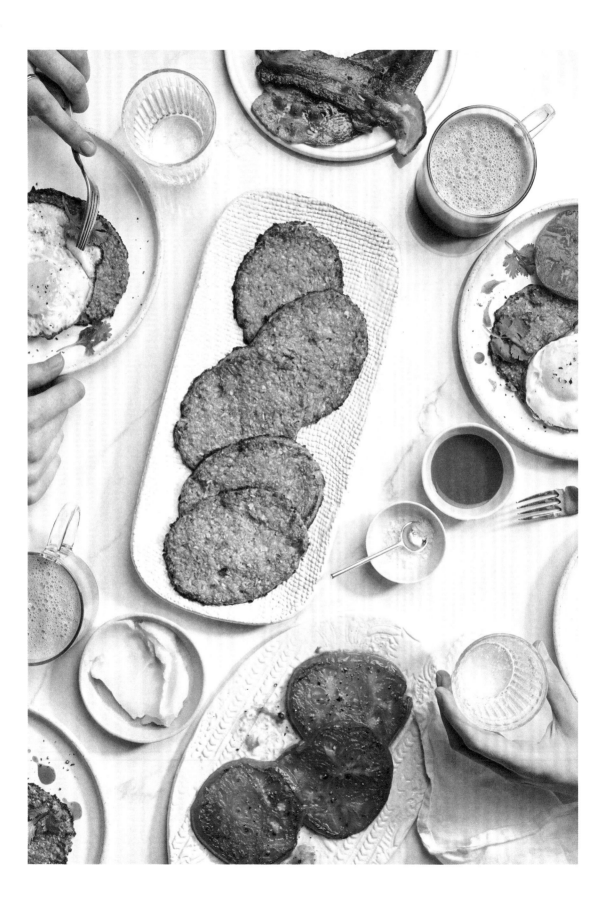

Gluten-Free ◆ Grain-Free ◆ Nut-Free ◆ Keto-Friendly ◆
Paleo-Friendly ◆ Vegetarian Option ◆ *Serves 2 to 4*

◆ Cheesy Cauliflower Hash Browns

This recipe came about as I was experimenting with how to make cauliflower into pizza crust. I was so impressed by how the cheese and eggs helped the cauliflower stick together that I figured the batter would make perfect hash browns. The verdict? They are utterly delicious! You can serve them with bacon and eggs for a leisurely weekend breakfast, alongside some sliced tomato and avocado for extra fibre.

1 large head of cauliflower, roughly chopped

½ cup (125 mL) grated pecorino cheese

2 tablespoons (30 mL) ghee or Plain Jane Ghee (page 271), at room temperature

2 pasture-raised or organic eggs

1 teaspoon (5 mL) garlic powder

1 teaspoon (5 mL) sweet paprika

1 teaspoon (5 mL) sea salt

To Serve

4 Ghee-Fried Eggs (page 269)

4 slices of Perfect Oven Bacon (page 270)

1 tomato, sliced

1 avocado, peeled, pitted, and sliced

1. Position racks in the upper and lower thirds of the oven. Preheat the oven to 425°F (220°C). Line 2 baking sheets with parchment paper.

2. In a food processor on high speed, process the cauliflower until coarsely ground. Wrap the cauliflower in a clean kitchen towel and squeeze to remove as much liquid as possible.

3. Transfer the cauliflower to a large bowl. Add the pecorino, ghee, eggs, garlic powder, paprika, and salt. Stir to combine.

4. Divide the mixture into 8 portions and shape them into ½-inch (1 cm) thick hash browns on the prepared baking sheets. Bake until the edges are golden brown, 25 to 30 minutes. (You do not need to flip the hash browns.) Let cool for 10 minutes to help the hash browns stick together.

5. Serve on a platter, alongside Ghee-Fried Eggs, Perfect Oven Bacon, and sliced tomato and avocado.

◆ **Vegetarian:** Skip the bacon.

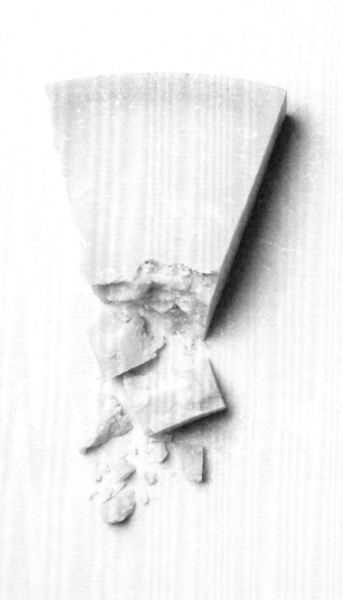

Soups and Salads

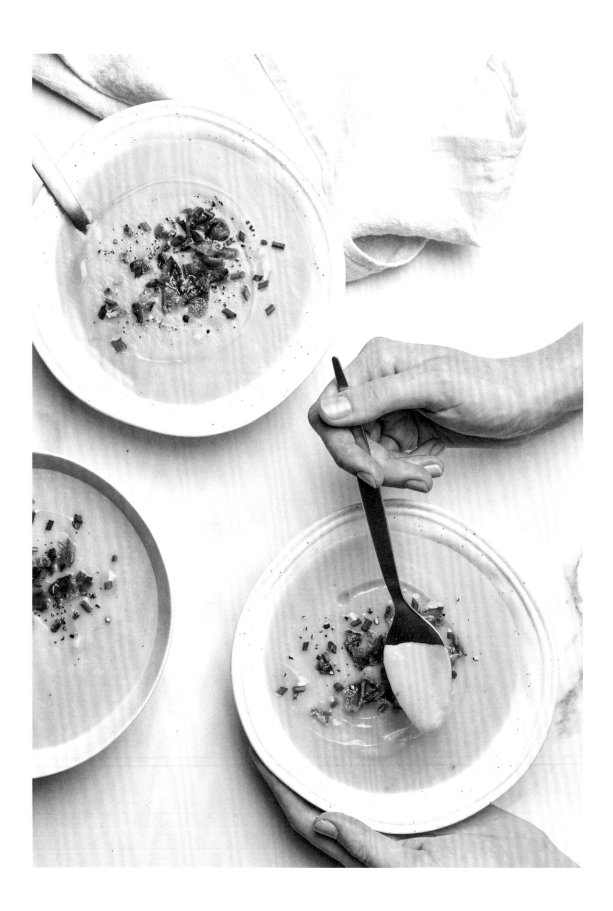

Potato and Leek Soup with Bacon Bits

This is a delicious version of a classic potato and leek soup, which I always have in my rotation during the fall and winter. I use a combination of bacon fat and ghee to make the soup super creamy and flavourful, without the use of heavy cream. The crunchy bits of bacon and a drizzle of good-quality extra-virgin olive oil on top make this soup irresistible.

4 slices organic bacon

2 tablespoons (30 mL) ghee or Plain Jane Ghee (page 271)

2 large leeks (white and light green parts only), roughly chopped

3 medium russet potatoes, peeled and chopped

4 cups (1 L) seasoned organic chicken broth or Chicken Bone Broth (page 272)

¾ teaspoon (4 mL) sea salt

Pinch of nutmeg

To Serve

Chopped fresh chives (optional)

Extra-virgin olive oil, to drizzle

1. In a large Dutch oven or a heavy-bottomed pot with a tight-fitting lid over medium heat, cook the bacon, flipping occasionally, until crispy, 18 to 20 minutes. Using tongs, transfer the bacon to a plate lined with paper towel to absorb excess oil. Leave the bacon fat in the pan.

2. Add the ghee, leeks, and potatoes and cook, stirring occasionally, until the leeks start to turn golden brown, 5 to 7 minutes.

3. Add the chicken broth and bring to a boil over high heat. Reduce the heat to medium and simmer, covered, until the potatoes are fork-tender, 10 to 12 minutes. Remove from the heat.

4. Using an immersion blender or a high-speed blender, purée the soup until smooth. Add the salt and nutmeg. Stir to combine.

5. To serve, crumble the bacon into small pieces. Divide the soup among bowls and top with bacon bits and chives, if using. Drizzle with olive oil. Store leftover soup in an airtight container in the fridge for up to 3 days.

Dairy-Free ◆ Gluten-Free Option ◆ Grain-Free Option
◆ Nut-Free ◆ Paleo-Friendly Option ◆ *Serves 4*

Creamy Tomato Soup with Garlic Sourdough Croutons

This recipe is a simple, fat-fuelled version of tomato soup, seasoned with Spanish-inspired flavours. It is creamy and satisfying, as all tomato soup should be. I use coconut cream and ghee in place of heavy cream and butter, which adds creaminess without all the dairy. To balance the flavours, I add a touch of maple syrup and apple cider vinegar, which takes this soup to the next level. Our recipe testers loved the garlic croutons so much that I made sure to include some extra croutons for snacking on before your guests arrive (trust me, you'll want to!).

Creamy Tomato Soup

3 tablespoons (45 mL) ghee or Plain Jane Ghee (page 271)

1 medium yellow onion, diced

2 cloves garlic, minced

1 teaspoon (5 mL) sweet paprika

2 teaspoons (10 mL) fresh thyme leaves

¼ teaspoon (1 mL) red chili flakes

¼ cup (60 mL) tomato paste

1 can (28 ounces/796 mL) whole or crushed tomatoes

1 teaspoon (5 mL) pure maple syrup

3 cups (750 mL) seasoned organic chicken broth or Chicken Bone Broth (page 272)

½ cup (125 mL) coconut cream, skimmed from 1 can (14 ounces/400 mL) full-fat coconut milk, refrigerated overnight

½ teaspoon (2 mL) apple cider vinegar

Sea salt and black pepper, to taste

Garlic Sourdough Croutons (makes a few extra)

3 tablespoons (45 mL) ghee or Plain Jane Ghee (page 271), at room temperature

3 large slices of crusty sourdough bread, cut into bite-size cubes

3 cloves garlic, minced

Sea salt, to taste

1. **Make the Creamy Tomato Soup** In a large Dutch oven or a heavy-bottomed pot with a tight-fitting lid over medium heat, melt the ghee. Add the onion and cook, stirring occasionally, until softened, 7 to 8 minutes. Add the garlic, paprika, thyme, and chili flakes and cook until fragrant, about 1 minute.

2. Add the tomato paste and stir to combine. Cook, stirring constantly, until the paste has darkened slightly, 2 to 3 minutes. Add the canned tomatoes, maple syrup, and chicken broth. Bring to a boil, then reduce the heat to medium and simmer, uncovered, stirring occasionally, for 40 minutes.

3. Add the coconut cream and apple cider vinegar. Using an immersion blender or a high-speed blender, purée the soup until smooth. Season with salt and pepper. Over medium heat, simmer, uncovered, for 8 minutes.

4. **Meanwhile, Make the Garlic Sourdough Croutons** In a large cast-iron skillet over medium-high heat, melt the ghee. When the pan is hot, add the bread cubes in a single layer. Fry until crispy and golden brown, 2 to 3 minutes per side. Stir in the garlic and cook for 30 more seconds. Sprinkle with salt.

5. To serve, divide the soup among bowls and top with the croutons. Store leftover soup in an airtight container in the fridge for up to 3 days.

- **Gluten-Free:** Use gluten-free bread instead of sourdough bread.
  Grain-Free and Paleo-Friendly: Skip the Garlic Sourdough Croutons.

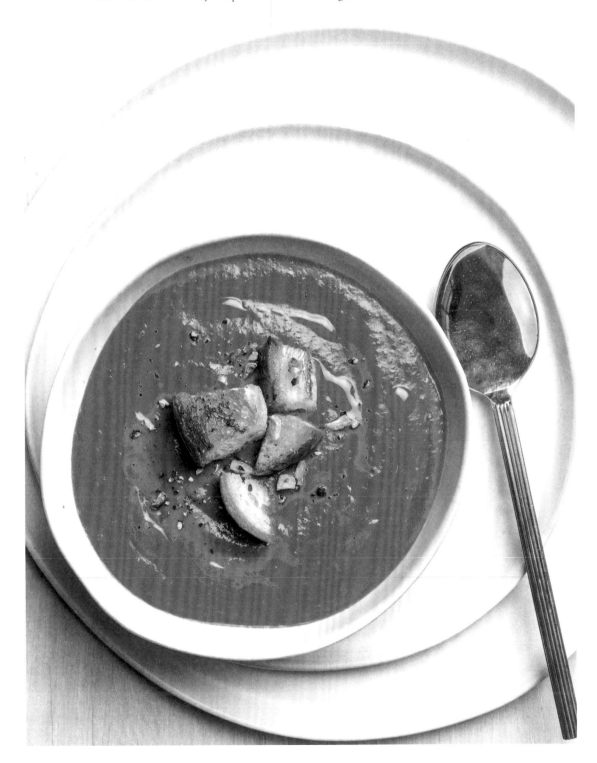

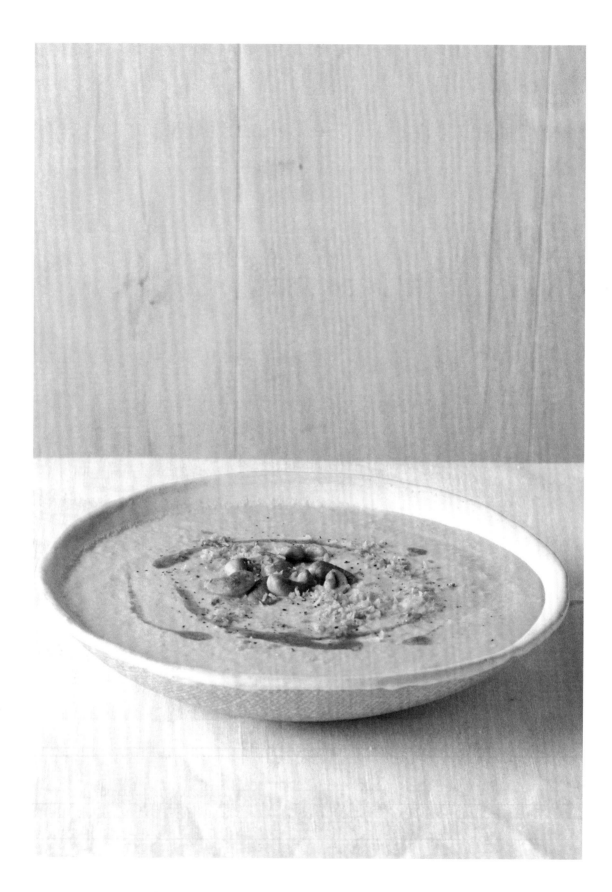

Dairy-Free ◆ Gluten-Free ◆ Grain-Free ◆ Keto-Friendly
◆ Paleo-Friendly ◆ Vegan Option ◆ Vegetarian ◆ *Serves 4 to 6*

Turmeric Lemon Soup with Ghee-Fried Cashews

When I first met my husband, he made this comforting soup for me, and it won my heart instantly. It has a vibrant yellow colour, lemony fresh flavour, and creamy texture—it's like happiness in a bowl. We have since adapted the recipe together, making it more nutrient dense. If you do not own a high-speed blender, you can soak the cashews for 15 minutes in hot water, drain them, and then process the soup in a standard blender.

Turmeric Lemon Soup

3 tablespoons (45 mL) ghee or Plain Jane Ghee (page 271)

1 medium yellow onion, diced

1 yellow bell pepper, diced

½ head of cauliflower, roughly chopped

1 cup (250 mL) raw cashews

2½ cups (625 mL) seasoned organic vegetable broth, more as needed

½ cup (125 mL) coconut cream, skimmed from 1 can (14 ounces/400 mL) full-fat coconut milk, refrigerated overnight

¼ cup (60 mL) fresh lemon juice

¼ cup (60 mL) nutritional yeast

½ teaspoon (2 mL) ground turmeric

½ teaspoon (2 mL) sea salt

¼ teaspoon (1 mL) chili powder

Ghee-Fried Cashews

1 tablespoon (15 mL) ghee or Plain Jane Ghee (page 271)

⅓ cup (75 mL) raw cashews

½ teaspoon (2 mL) ground turmeric

1. **Make the Turmeric Lemon Soup** In a large Dutch oven or a heavy-bottomed pot with a tight-fitting lid over medium-high heat, melt the ghee. Add the onion and bell pepper and sauté, stirring occasionally, until softened, 5 to 7 minutes.

2. Add the cauliflower, cashews, vegetable broth, coconut cream, lemon juice, nutritional yeast, turmeric, salt, and chili powder. Bring to a boil, then reduce the heat to medium and simmer, covered, until the cauliflower is fork-tender, 10 to 12 minutes.

3. Transfer the soup to a high-speed blender. Blend on high speed until smooth. Add ½ cup (125 mL) more broth, as needed, to thin the soup to desired consistency.

4. **Make the Ghee-Fried Cashews** In a medium skillet over medium heat, melt the ghee. Add the cashews and turmeric. Stir to combine, then cook, stirring occasionally, until the cashews are golden brown, 2 to 3 minutes.

5. To serve, divide the soup among bowls. Garnish with Ghee-Fried Cashews and a drizzle of ghee from the pan. Store leftover soup in an airtight container in the fridge for up to 3 days.

◆ **Vegan:** Use virgin coconut oil instead of ghee.

Dairy-Free ◆ Gluten-Free ◆ Grain-Free ◆ Keto-Friendly Option
◆ Nut-Free ◆ Paleo-Friendly Option ◆ *Serves 4 to 6*

Restorative Kimchi and Pork Soup

This nourishing recipe is inspired by the famous Korean soup called *kimchi-jjigae*. I first made this soup when I was looking for ways to use kimchi after getting a large batch from a Korean friend. I turn to it when I feel under the weather and crave something comforting and warm. The browned pork and toasted sesame oil meld to create an irresistible flavour. I make a point to gently stir in the kimchi right at the end to preserve its beneficial bacteria, which further add to the soup's restorative value. To make it into a more substantial meal, serve over rice or soba noodles.

1 tablespoon (15 mL) ghee, Plain Jane Ghee (page 271), or avocado oil

1 pound (450 g) organic ground pork

½ small yellow onion, thinly sliced

3 cloves garlic, minced

1 (1-inch/2.5 cm) piece of fresh ginger, peeled and minced

4 cups (1 L) seasoned organic chicken broth or Chicken Bone Broth (page 272)

3 tablespoons (45 mL) gluten-free tamari or coconut aminos

8 ounces (225 g) organic silken tofu, cut into ½-inch (1 cm) cubes

2 large shiitake mushrooms, cleaned, trimmed, and sliced into quarters

2 tablespoons (30 mL) sesame seeds

2 cups (500 mL) kimchi, roughly chopped

To Serve

Toasted sesame oil

Sliced green onions (white and light green parts only)

1. In a large Dutch oven or a heavy-bottomed pot with a tight-fitting lid over medium-high heat, melt the ghee. Add the ground pork and cook, stirring often and breaking up large pieces, until browned, 2 to 3 minutes.

2. Add the onion, garlic, and ginger and cook, stirring frequently, for 1 minute. Add the chicken broth, tamari, tofu, and mushrooms. Cover and bring to a boil, then reduce the heat to medium-low and simmer for 10 to 15 minutes, stirring occasionally.

3. Meanwhile, heat a dry, medium skillet over medium heat. Add the sesame seeds in a single layer and toast, stirring occasionally, until fragrant and lightly browned, 4 to 5 minutes.

4. Remove the soup from the heat and gently stir in the kimchi.

5. To serve, ladle the soup into bowls. Top with a drizzle of toasted sesame oil. Garnish with green onions and toasted sesame seeds. Store leftover soup in an airtight container in the fridge for up to 3 days.

◆ **Keto-Friendly and Paleo-Friendly:** Omit the tofu and use coconut aminos instead of gluten-free tamari.

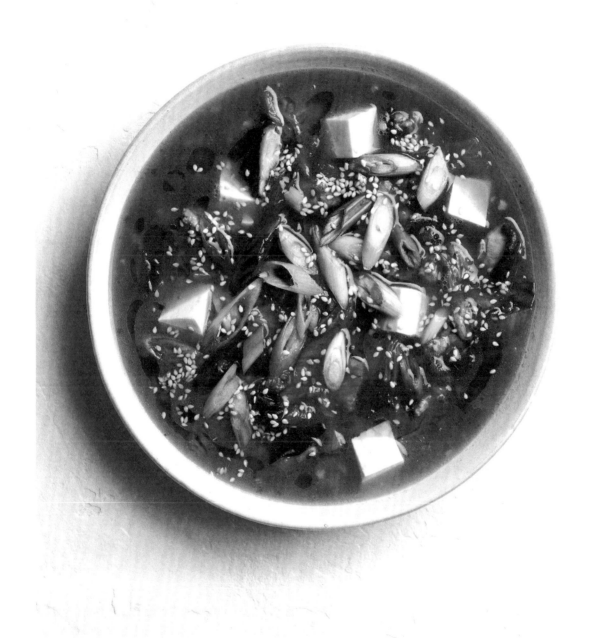

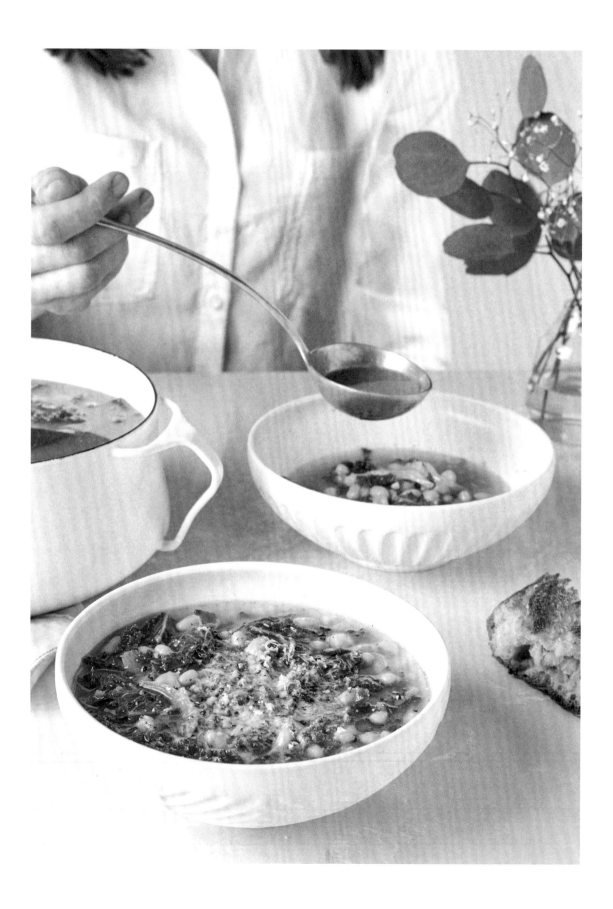

◆ Garlicky White Bean, Kale, and Pesto Soup

This is a great soup for a light weeknight supper, slurped up with some crusty whole-grain sourdough bread. The soup comes together rather quickly on the stove, but most of the deeper flavours and nutrients come from homemade Chicken Bone Broth (page 272) and Fresh Pesto (page 276). You can save a lot of time by using store-bought chicken broth and pesto, but you might lose some of the depth of flavour.

2 tablespoons (30 mL) ghee or Plain Jane Ghee (page 271)

1 medium yellow onion, thinly sliced

3 cloves garlic, minced

6 cups (1.5 L) seasoned organic chicken broth or Chicken Bone Broth (page 272)

2 cans (14 ounces/400 mL each) navy beans, drained and rinsed

1 small bunch of curly green kale, stems and ribs removed, leaves chopped (about 6 cups/1.5 L)

1 teaspoon (5 mL) sea salt

½ teaspoon (2 mL) black pepper

To Serve

½ cup (125 mL) Fresh Pesto (page 276) or store-bought pesto

¼ cup (60 mL) grated pecorino cheese

Crusty, whole-grain sourdough bread

1. In a large Dutch oven or a heavy-bottomed pot with a tight-fitting lid over medium heat, melt the ghee. Add the onion and cook, stirring occasionally, until softened, 7 to 8 minutes. Add the garlic and cook for 1 minute.

2. Add the chicken broth and navy beans. Bring to a boil, then reduce the heat to medium-low.

3. Stir in the kale and simmer until the kale is wilted, 1 to 2 minutes. Add the salt and pepper.

4. Just before serving, gently stir in the pesto. Ladle the soup into bowls and top with grated cheese. Serve with crusty bread. Store leftover soup in an airtight container in the fridge for up to 3 days.

◆ **Gluten-Free:** Serve with gluten-free bread instead of whole-grain sourdough bread.

Green Gazpacho with Avocado and Citrus

This green gazpacho is a cold soup that is instantly refreshing on hot days. The good fats from the avocado, hemp seeds, and olive oil make it creamy, substantial, and filling, while the citrus notes from the grapefruit and lime juice add freshness and acidity to balance the flavours. The soup is made in a blender or food processor, so it comes together in a matter of minutes. A word to the wise: this soup is best enjoyed immediately, as the avocado will brown over time.

2 large avocados, peeled and pitted

1 grapefruit, peeled, white pith and seeds removed

1 cup (250 mL) peeled and diced English cucumber, more to garnish

2 tablespoons (30 mL) freshly squeezed lime juice

2 cups (500 mL) packed baby spinach

1 cup (250 mL) packed fresh basil leaves

2 tablespoons (30 mL) hulled hemp seeds, more to garnish

2 teaspoons (10 mL) pure maple syrup

1 teaspoon (5 mL) sea salt

½ teaspoon (2 mL) black pepper

1 cup (250 mL) water, more as needed

6 ice cubes

Extra-virgin olive oil, to drizzle

1. In a high-speed blender or a food processor, add the avocado, grapefruit, cucumber, lime juice, baby spinach, basil, hemp seeds, maple syrup, salt, pepper, water, and ice cubes. Blend on high speed until smooth, about 30 seconds. Add more water, as needed, to thin the soup to desired consistency.

2. To serve, divide the soup among bowls and drizzle with olive oil. Garnish with diced cucumber and a sprinkle of hemp seeds. Serve immediately.

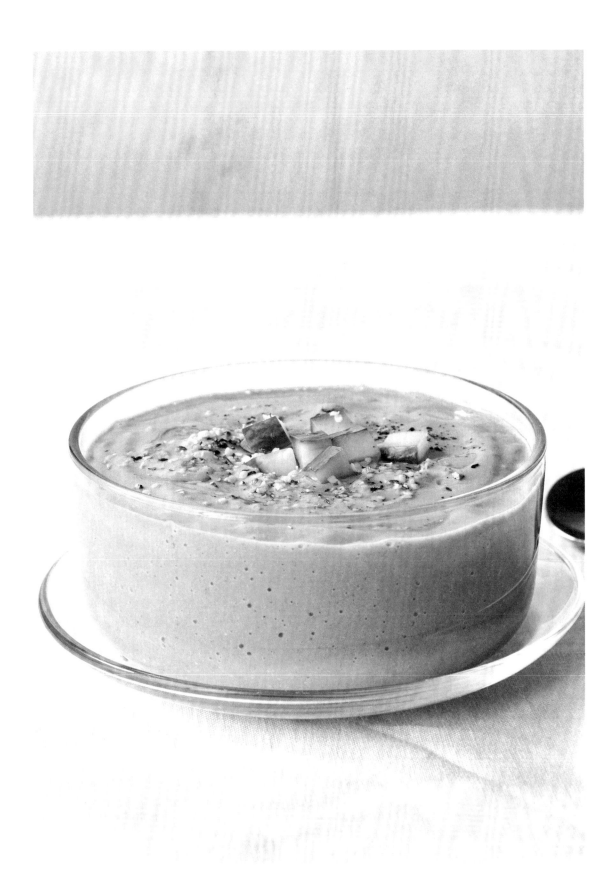

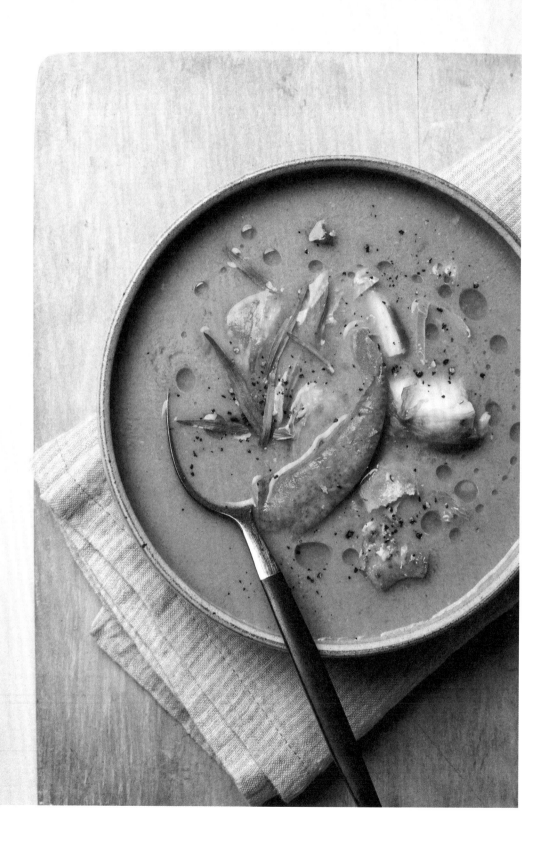

Dairy-Free ◆ Gluten-Free ◆ Grain-Free ◆ Nut-Free ◆ *Serves 4 to 6 as a side*

Lobster and Wild Salmon Bisque

This lobster bisque is creamy, velvety, and delicious. Lobsters are a great source of omega-3 fats EPA and DHA, which support brain and heart health. The key to making bisque is to slowly simmer the lobster shells with aromatics until you have a really flavourful stock. This gives the stock a depth of flavour you simply can't get from store-bought varieties. Ask for lobster shells and meat at a good fishmonger. This is much more convenient than buying whole lobsters. You'll save money and avoid making a mess!

2 tablespoons (30 mL) ghee or Plain Jane Ghee (page 271)

1 medium yellow onion, diced

1 stalk celery, diced

1 carrot, peeled and diced

2 cloves garlic, minced

¾ cup (175 mL) dry white wine

6 cups (1.5 L) water

2 lobster shells, fresh or frozen, chopped into 2-inch (5 cm) pieces

2 bay leaves

6 black peppercorns

5 sprigs fresh tarragon

1 tablespoon (15 mL) arrowroot starch

¼ cup (60 mL) tomato paste

1 cup (250 mL) coconut cream, skimmed from 1 can (14 ounces/400 mL) full-fat coconut milk, refrigerated overnight

2 teaspoons (10 mL) sea salt

12 ounces (340 g) fresh or thawed frozen lobster meat, roughly chopped

8 ounces (225 g) skin-on wild salmon fillet, roughly chopped

To Serve

Fresh tarragon leaves

Extra-virgin olive oil

Freshly ground black pepper

1. In a large Dutch oven or a heavy-bottomed pot with a tight-fitting lid over medium-high heat, melt the ghee. Add the onion, celery, and carrots. Cook, uncovered, stirring occasionally, until the onion is softened and golden brown, 7 to 8 minutes. Add the garlic and cook for 1 minute.

2. Add the white wine and cook, uncovered, until most of the wine has evaporated, 3 to 4 minutes.

3. Add the water, lobster shells, bay leaves, peppercorns, and tarragon. Bring to a boil, then reduce the heat to medium and simmer, covered, for 35 to 40 minutes. Strain the broth through a large fine mesh strainer set over a large heat-proof bowl. Discard the solids.

4. In a small bowl, combine the arrowroot starch and 3 tablespoons (45 mL) of the strained broth. Whisk until completely smooth. Add the starch mixture to the broth and whisk to combine. Add the tomato paste, coconut cream, and salt, whisking to combine.

5. Return the broth mixture to the pot and bring to a boil over high heat. Reduce the heat to medium and simmer, uncovered, stirring occasionally, until the broth has thickened and reduced by a quarter, 12 to 15 minutes. Remove from the heat.

6. Add the lobster meat and wild salmon to the broth. Stir to combine. Let sit, covered, for 5 minutes (the residual heat will warm the lobster and gently cook the salmon).

7. Ladle the bisque into bowls and garnish with fresh tarragon. Drizzle with olive oil and finish with a sprinkle of pepper.

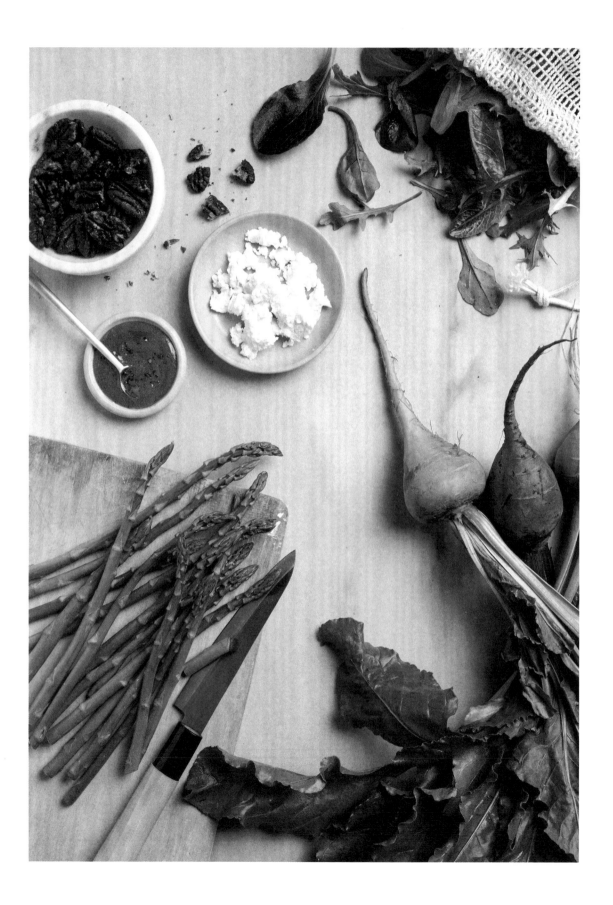

Country Salad with Candied Pecans and Goat Cheese

This country salad combines the earthy sweetness of roasted beets with the creaminess of goat cheese and the crunchiness of pecans and pumpkin seeds. The candied pecans are so addictive that I included extra for snacking on (trust me, you'll want to!). The beets take time to roast, but it really concentrates their sweetness and makes them flavourful. While the beets are in the oven, you can make the candied pecans and asparagus. This is a perfect rustic salad to enjoy with roasted chicken or any simply grilled protein.

Country Salad

2 medium red beets, scrubbed

1 tablespoon (15 mL) + ½ teaspoon (2 mL) avocado oil, divided

1 bunch of thin asparagus, ends trimmed and sliced on the diagonal into 2-inch (5 cm) pieces

6 cups (1.5 L) loosely packed spring mix (about 5 ounces/140 g)

3½ ounces (100 g) goat cheese, crumbled (optional)

½ cup (125 mL) raw pumpkin seeds

Candied Pecans (makes extra)

2 cups (500 mL) raw pecans

2 teaspoons (10 mL) coconut sugar

½ teaspoon (2 mL) cinnamon

½ teaspoon (2 mL) sea salt

2 tablespoons (30 mL) pure maple syrup

2 teaspoons (10 mL) melted ghee or Plain Jane Ghee (page 271)

Balsamic Mustard Vinaigrette

¼ cup (60 mL) extra-virgin olive oil

2 tablespoons (30 mL) balsamic vinegar

2 teaspoons (10 mL) Dijon mustard

1 small clove garlic, grated

Sea salt and black pepper, to taste

1. Position racks in the upper and lower thirds of the oven. Preheat the oven to 400°F (200°C). Line 2 baking sheets with parchment paper.

2. **Roast the Beets** Rub each beet with ¼ teaspoon (1 mL) of the avocado oil and place them on a prepared baking sheet. Roast until fork-tender, 40 to 60 minutes. When the beets are cool to the touch, peel off the skins. Slice the beets into ¼-inch (5 mm) thick half-moons.

3. **Meanwhile, Make the Candied Pecans** In a medium bowl, add the pecans, coconut sugar, cinnamon, and salt. Stir to combine. Add the maple syrup and melted ghee. Stir again to combine.

4. Arrange the pecans in a single layer on the second prepared baking sheet. Roast until the pecans are caramelized and sticky, 7 to 9 minutes. Remove from the oven and let cool for 10 minutes to allow them to harden.

5. **Cook the Asparagus** In a large skillet over medium-high heat, heat the remaining 1 tablespoon (15 mL) avocado oil. Add the asparagus and sauté, stirring occasionally, until tender, 4 to 6 minutes.

recipe continues

recipe continued

6. **Make the Balsamic Mustard Vinaigrette** In a small bowl, whisk together the olive oil, balsamic vinegar, mustard, garlic, salt, and pepper.

7. Add the spring mix to a large salad bowl. Top with 1 cup (250 mL) of the Candied Pecans, roasted beets, asparagus, goat cheese (if using), and pumpkin seeds. Just before serving, add the Balsamic Mustard Vinaigrette and toss to combine.

◆ **Paleo-Friendly:** Substitute 1 diced avocado for the goat cheese.
Vegan: Use virgin coconut oil instead of ghee to roast the pecans. Substitute 1 diced avocado for the goat cheese.

Chicken Cobb Salad with Jammy Eggs

This salad makes for a great lunch and can hold its own as a complete meal because it is just so filling and satisfying. I use cheese, Jammy Eggs (page 269), and avocado for healthy fats and protein, while the lemony mustard dressing adds acidity and sharpness to balance out the richness. Roquefort is a sheep's milk blue cheese, which is easier to digest than cow's milk blue cheese. If you don't like blue cheese or avoid dairy, just leave it out—the salad will still be delicious!

Chicken Cobb Salad

2 skinless, boneless organic chicken breasts (7½ ounces/ 214 g each)

1 tablespoon (15 mL) avocado oil

Sea salt and black pepper, to taste

1 head of butter lettuce, leaves separated, washed, and torn

½ pound (225 g) Perfect Oven Bacon (page 270), sliced into bite-size pieces

4 Jammy Eggs (page 269), sliced in half

3½ ounces (100 g) Roquefort blue cheese, crumbled (optional)

1 large heirloom tomato, sliced into wedges

1 avocado, peeled, pitted, and cut into wedges

Mustard Lemon Vinaigrette

½ cup (125 mL) extra-virgin olive oil

¼ cup (60 mL) fresh lemon juice

1 small clove garlic, grated

2 teaspoons (10 mL) Dijon mustard

½ teaspoon (2 mL) sea salt

¼ teaspoon (1 mL) black pepper

1. Preheat the oven to 425°F (220°C). Line a baking sheet with parchment paper.

2. **Roast the Chicken Breasts** In a medium bowl, toss the chicken breasts with the avocado oil, salt, and pepper. Place the chicken breasts on the prepared baking sheet and roast until the internal temperature reaches 165°F (75°C), 25 to 30 minutes, turning them halfway through roasting time. Remove from the oven and let the chicken rest for 10 minutes. Using 2 forks, shred into bite-size pieces.

3. **Make the Mustard Lemon Vinaigrette** In a small bowl, whisk together the olive oil, lemon juice, garlic, mustard, salt, and pepper.

4. **Assemble the Salad** Place the lettuce leaves on a large serving platter. Drizzle half of the Mustard Lemon Vinaigrette over the lettuce.

5. Arrange the shredded chicken, bacon pieces, Jammy Eggs, blue cheese (if using), tomato, and avocado on top of the lettuce. Drizzle the remaining vinaigrette over the salad.

◆ **Dairy-Free:** Skip the blue cheese.

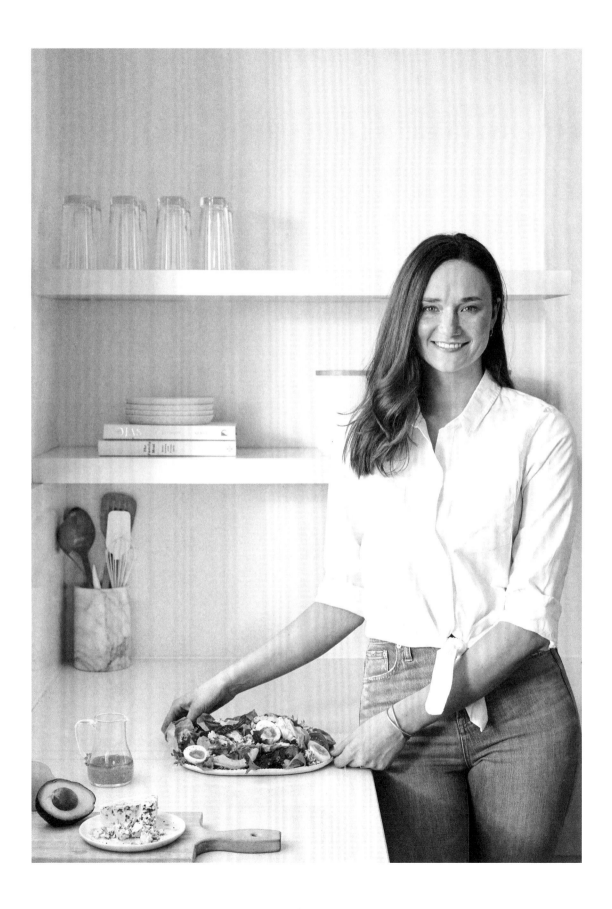

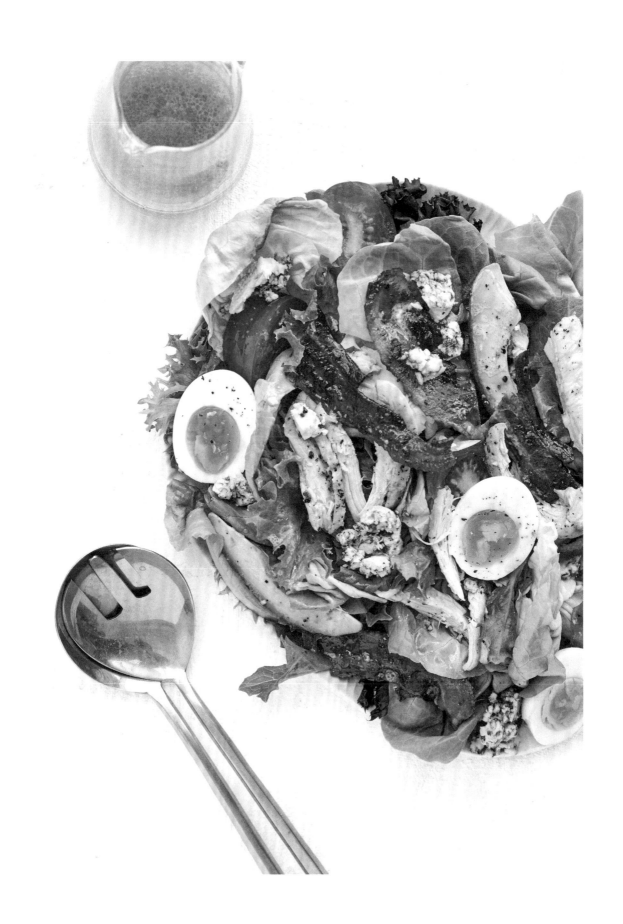

Warm Quinoa Salad with Fried Halloumi and Bacon

A quinoa salad to trump all other quinoa salads! I am the last person in the world who you will find eating a cold, depressing quinoa salad for lunch—it just feels like I am depriving myself too much. So, I decided to create this warm, hearty version, which is full of healthy fats and will not leave you feeling hungry. Each bite feels like a treat, with salty bits of halloumi and bacon, crunchy walnuts, and crisp apple, all tossed in a fresh lemony dressing. Walnuts are high in fibre and healthy fats, which makes them a great addition.

Warm Quinoa Salad

1¼ cups (300 mL) quinoa, rinsed and drained

2 cups (500 mL) seasoned organic chicken broth or Chicken Bone Broth (page 272)

⅓ pound (150 g) halloumi cheese, preferably sheep's milk

1 cup (250 mL) raw walnuts

6 slices of Perfect Oven Bacon (page 270), cut into bite-size pieces

1 red apple (Gala, Fuji, or Honeycrisp), cored and chopped into bite-size pieces

2 cups (500 mL) tightly packed baby arugula or baby spinach

1 tablespoon (15 mL) hulled hemp seeds

Honey Lemon Dressing

¼ cup (60 mL) extra-virgin olive oil

2 tablespoons (30 mL) fresh lemon juice

1 tablespoon (15 mL) raw liquid honey

1 teaspoon (5 mL) lemon zest

Pinch of freshly ground black pepper

1. **Cook the Quinoa** In a medium saucepan over high heat, bring the quinoa and chicken broth to a boil. Reduce the heat to low and cook, covered, until all of the broth has been absorbed, 12 to 15 minutes. Remove from the heat and fluff with a fork. Cover to keep warm.

2. **Fry the Halloumi** Slice the halloumi into ¼-inch (5 mm) thick slices, then cut each slice in half again. Heat a medium skillet over medium-high heat. Lay the halloumi slices in the pan and cook until golden brown, 1 to 2 minutes per side. Transfer to a plate.

3. Reduce the heat to medium. In the same skillet (no need to wipe the pan), toast the walnuts, stirring often, until fragrant and browned, 3 to 5 minutes. Remove from the pan and let cool. Roughly chop.

4. **Make the Honey Lemon Dressing** In a small bowl, whisk together the olive oil, lemon juice, honey, lemon zest, and pepper.

5. **Assemble the Salad** In a large bowl, combine the quinoa, halloumi, walnuts, bacon, apple, arugula, and hemp seeds. Toss with the Honey Lemon Dressing. Serve warm.

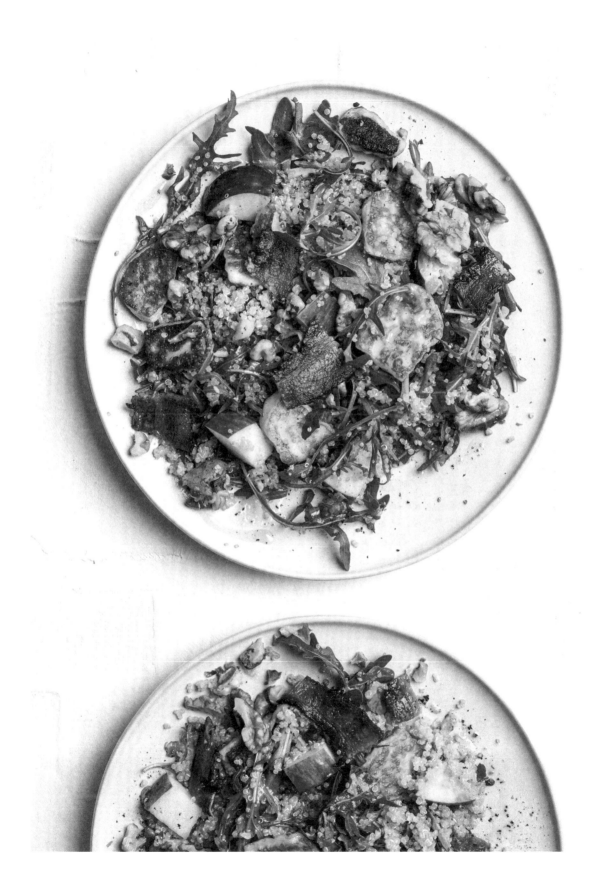

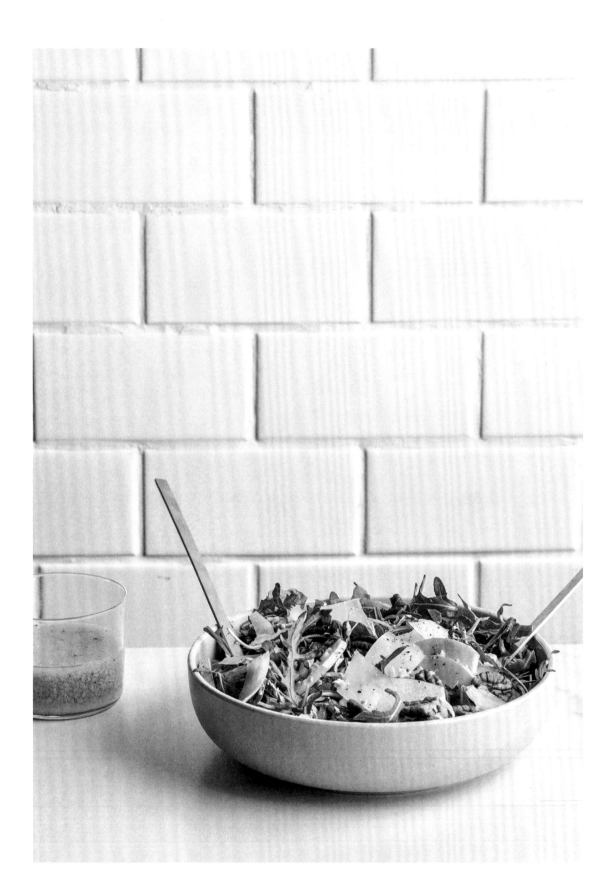

Gluten-Free ◆ Grain-Free ◆ Vegetarian ◆ *Serves 4 to 6 as a side*

Avocado Rocket Salad with Mustard Lemon Vinaigrette

This simple, elevated salad is delicious served alongside any protein, such as my Pan Seared Grass-Fed Steaks with Crispy Roasted Potatoes (page 127). Peppery arugula is tossed with crunchy pecans, creamy avocado, crisp Asian pear, and shaved Brussels sprouts to create the perfect balance of flavours and textures. I often make this salad because it is quick to assemble and goes with everything. It has a variety of healthy fats from sheep's milk cheese, avocado, pecans, and sunflower seeds.

Mustard Lemon Vinaigrette

¼ cup (60 mL) extra-virgin olive oil

2 tablespoons (30 mL) fresh lemon juice

1 teaspoon (5 mL) Dijon mustard

¼ teaspoon (1 mL) sea salt

Pinch of black pepper

Avocado Rocket Salad

6 Brussels sprouts, ends trimmed, tough outer leaves removed, and cut in half

6 cups (1.5 L) loosely packed baby arugula (about 5 ounces/ 140 g)

1 avocado, peeled, pitted, and diced

2 ounces (55 g) pecorino cheese, shaved into large pieces with a vegetable peeler

1 firm-ripe Asian pear, halved, cored, and thinly sliced

1 cup (250 mL) raw pecans

¼ cup (60 mL) raw sunflower seeds

1. **Make the Mustard Lemon Vinaigrette** In a small bowl, whisk together the olive oil, lemon juice, mustard, salt, and pepper.
2. **Make the Avocado Rocket Salad** Using a sharp knife or a mandoline, carefully slice the Brussels sprouts as thinly as possible.
3. Add the arugula to a large salad bowl. Top with the Brussels sprouts, avocado, cheese, pear, pecans, and sunflower seeds. Just before serving, add the Mustard Lemon Vinaigrette and toss to combine.

Chopped Avocado Caprese Salad

This chopped salad is a real crowd-pleaser and only takes a few minutes to throw together. It makes for a great side dish for a summer lunch. Try to find heirloom tomatoes when they are in season, as this recipe really highlights their flavour. The avocado and hemp seeds add a healthy dose of monounsaturated and omega-3 fats to the salad, making it both satisfying and delicious!

Balsamic Vinaigrette

¼ cup (60 mL) extra-virgin olive oil

2 tablespoons (30 mL) balsamic vinegar

Sea salt and black pepper, to taste

Chopped Avocado Caprese Salad

3 large heirloom tomatoes, cut into 1-inch (2.5 cm) chunks

7 ounces (200 g) fresh bocconcini, drained and sliced in half

1 large avocado, peeled, pitted, and cut into 1-inch (2.5 cm) chunks

½ cup (125 mL) packed fresh basil leaves (large pieces torn)

1 tablespoon (15 mL) hulled hemp seeds

1. **Make the Balsamic Vinaigrette** In a small bowl, whisk together the olive oil, balsamic vinegar, salt, and pepper.

2. **Make the Chopped Avocado Caprese Salad** To serve, arrange the tomatoes, bocconcini, avocado, and basil on a medium serving platter. Drizzle the Balsamic Vinaigrette over the salad and sprinkle with the hemp seeds.

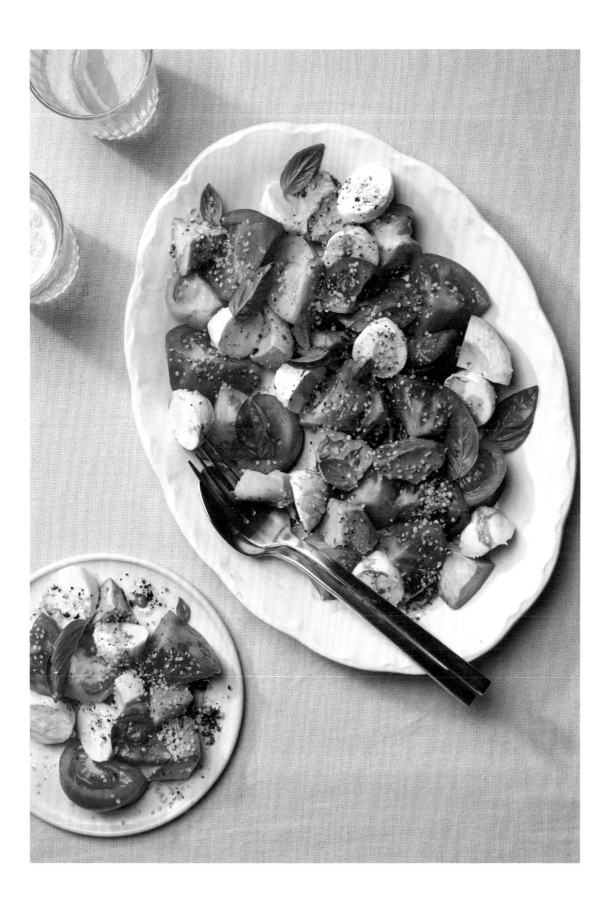

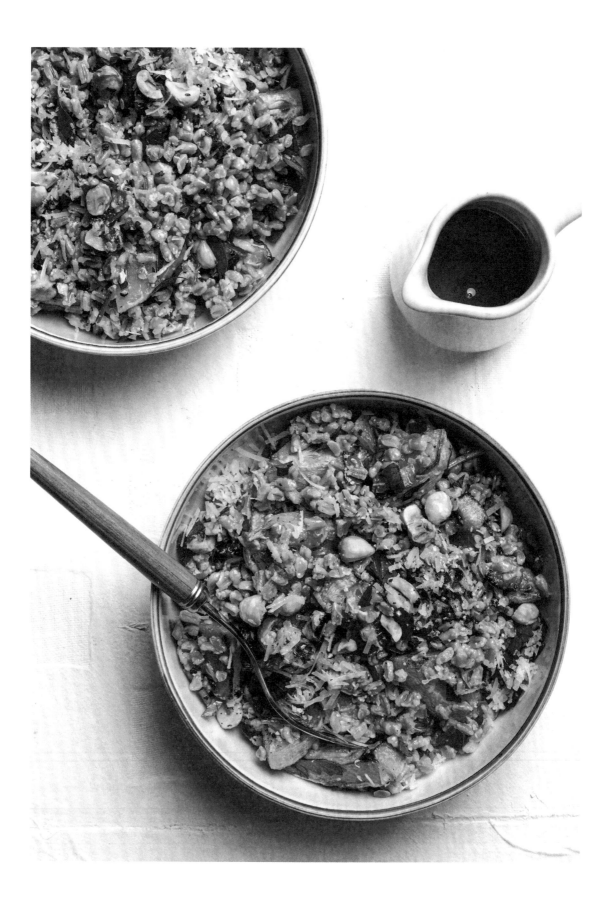

Warm Farro Salad with Hazelnuts and Pecorino

I am a sucker for a good grain salad, and I think this one is up there with the best of the autumn salads—balanced, filling, and healthy. It makes for a great side dish at Thanksgiving, and the leftovers are even better for lunch the next day! There are plenty of good fats from toasted hazelnuts, extra-virgin olive oil, and sheep's milk cheese, which make it very satisfying. Delicata squash is high in beta-carotene, which can help boost immunity during the colder months.

Farro Salad

2½ cups (625 mL) seasoned organic vegetable broth

2 cups (500 mL) farro, rinsed and drained

½ teaspoon (2 mL) sea salt, more to season

1 delicata squash, unpeeled and seeded

2 tablespoons (30 mL) avocado oil

Freshly ground black pepper, to taste

¾ cup (175 mL) raw hazelnuts

Apple Cider Vinaigrette

⅓ cup (75 mL) extra-virgin olive oil

3 tablespoons (45 mL) apple cider vinegar

1 tablespoon (15 mL) Dijon mustard

1 tablespoon (15 mL) raw honey or pure maple syrup

Sea salt and black pepper, to taste

To Serve

⅓ cup (75 mL) grated pecorino cheese

¼ cup (60 mL) loosely packed chopped fresh flat-leaf parsley

1. Preheat the oven to 450°F (230°C). Line a baking sheet with parchment paper.

2. In a medium saucepan over high heat, bring the vegetable broth to a boil. Add the farro and salt. Reduce to a simmer, cover, and cook until the farro is tender and chewy, 30 to 40 minutes. Remove from the heat and drain any excess liquid. Cover with a lid to keep warm.

3. **Meanwhile, Roast the Delicata Squash** Slice the squash into ½-inch (1 cm) thick slices, then cut each slice into bite-size pieces. In a medium bowl, toss the squash with the avocado oil and season with salt and pepper.

4. Arrange the squash in a single layer on the prepared baking sheet. Roast for 20 to 25 minutes, turning the squash halfway through baking time, until fork-tender.

5. **Toast the Hazelnuts** Heat a dry, large skillet over medium-high heat. Add the hazelnuts in a single layer and toast, tossing occasionally, until fragrant and browned, 5 to 6 minutes. Transfer to a cutting board to cool, then roughly chop the nuts into pieces.

6. **Make the Apple Cider Vinaigrette** In a small bowl, whisk together the olive oil, apple cider vinegar, mustard, honey, salt, and pepper.

7. In a large salad bowl, combine the cooked farro, squash, toasted hazelnuts, grated cheese, and parsley. Pour the Apple Cider Vinaigrette over the salad and toss to combine. Serve warm.

◆ **Dairy-Free and Vegan:** Skip the pecorino cheese.
   Nut-Free: Skip the hazelnuts.

Wild Salmon Niçoise with Jammy Eggs

This is a perfect weekday lunch that is simple to make and nutritious. Salmon, which has more omega-3 fatty acids and less mercury than tuna, gives a nice twist to the usual Niçoise salad. If you are in a hurry, you can save time by using leftover roasted salmon or substituting canned sockeye salmon. This salad has a fresh mustard vinaigrette that clings to the crisp butter lettuce just perfectly. Cook the Jammy Eggs (page 269) in a separate saucepan while the potatoes and green beans are cooking, and voilà—lunch is served!

Mustard Lemon Vinaigrette

½ cup (125 mL) extra-virgin olive oil

¼ cup (60 mL) fresh lemon juice

1 small clove garlic, grated

2 teaspoons (10 mL) Dijon mustard

½ teaspoon (2 mL) sea salt

¼ teaspoon (1 mL) pepper

Salad

1 pound (450 g) skin-on wild salmon fillet

Black pepper, to taste

1 tablespoon (15 mL) avocado oil

8 ounces (225 g) baby potatoes

1 tablespoon (15 mL) sea salt, more to season

7 ounces (200 g) green beans, ends trimmed

1 head of butter lettuce, leaves separated, washed, and torn

4 Jammy Eggs (page 269), sliced in half

1 medium heirloom tomato, sliced into wedges

¼ cup (60 mL) pitted Kalamata olives, cut in half

2 tablespoons (30 mL) drained capers

1. **Make the Mustard Lemon Vinaigrette** In a small bowl, whisk together the olive oil, lemon juice, garlic, mustard, salt, and pepper.

2. **Cook the Salmon** Season the salmon on both sides with salt and pepper. In a large skillet over medium-high heat, heat the avocado oil. Lay the salmon fillet, skin side down, in the pan. Reduce the heat to medium and cook until the skin is crispy, 3 to 5 minutes. Flip and cook for another 2 to 3 minutes, until the salmon is cooked all the way through.

3. Transfer the salmon to a cutting board. Using a fork, flake the salmon into bite-size pieces. Chop the crispy skin.

4. **Cook the Potatoes and Green Beans** Place the potatoes in a medium saucepan and fill with just enough water to cover them. Add the salt and bring to a boil over high heat. Cover and boil until fork-tender, 10 to 12 minutes. Using tongs, transfer the potatoes to a cutting board and slice them in half. Do not discard the water.

5. Add the green beans to the same saucepan and bring the water back to a boil over medium-high heat. Cover and blanch the beans until bright green and crisp-tender, 1 to 2 minutes. Using tongs, transfer the beans to a bowl of ice water, then drain.

6. To serve, arrange the lettuce on plates and drizzle with half of the Mustard Lemon Vinaigrette. Top with the flaked salmon, crispy salmon skin, green beans, potatoes, Jammy Eggs, tomato wedges, olives, and capers. Pour the remaining vinaigrette over top.

◆ **Keto-Friendly and Paleo-Friendly:** Skip the potatoes.

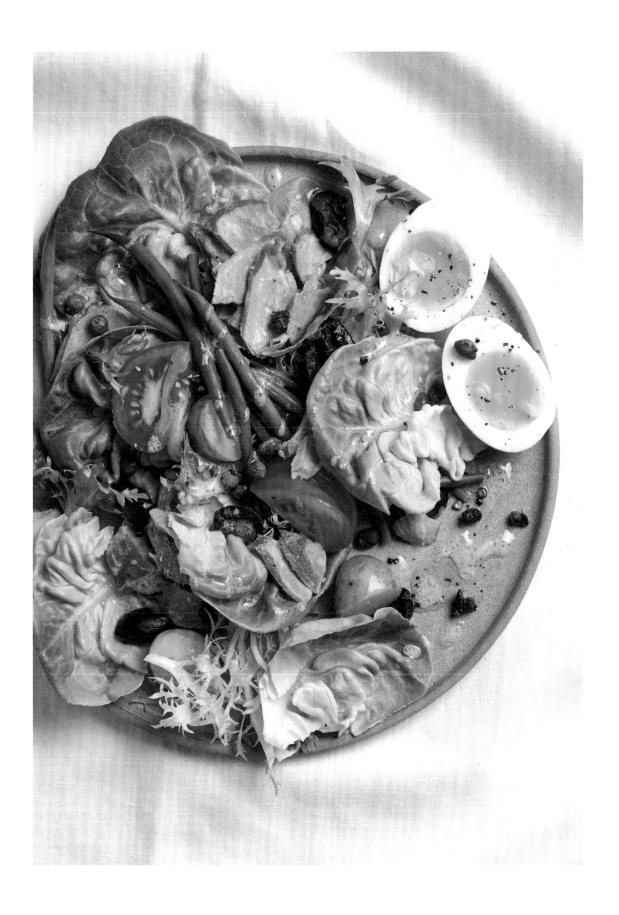

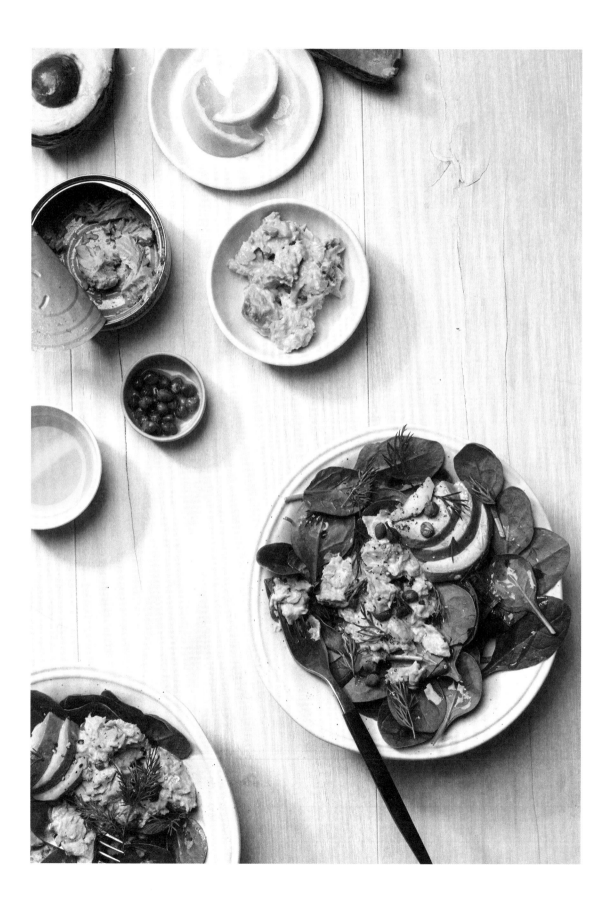

Easy Salmon Salad

I like to make this salad after a workout or whenever I want a light, healthy meal—especially in the summertime. It is served on a bed of baby spinach but is also delicious served as an open-faced sandwich. Canned salmon is a convenient source of omega-3 fatty acids, protein, and vitamin D. Look for canned salmon that comes with the bones and skin, as they contain most of the nutrients.

2 cans (5.3 ounces/150 g each) wild sockeye salmon, drained

⅓ cup (75 mL) Lemon Aioli (page 277)

4 cups (1 L) tightly packed baby spinach

1 tablespoon (15 mL) drained capers

½ cup (125 mL) chopped fresh dill

2 teaspoons (10 mL) extra-virgin olive oil

Pinch of flaky sea salt (optional)

1 avocado, peeled, pitted, and sliced

Fresh lemon wedges

1. In a small bowl, mix together the salmon and Lemon Aioli.
2. Divide the baby spinach among 4 bowls, then add a quarter of the salmon mixture to each bowl.
3. Top with the capers, dill, olive oil, and salt, if using. Serve with sliced avocado and lemon wedges.

Black Kale Salad with Smoked Trout and Hazelnuts

This is an epic salad! The omega-3-rich smoked trout really shines when tossed with the hearty kale, creamy avocado, tangy goat cheese, sharp radish, and toasted hazelnuts. Massaging the kale with olive oil and lemon juice helps the fibres break down and become easier to digest. Since this salad has plenty of healthy fats and protein, it can easily hold its own as a main. Having good-quality smoked trout can make a big difference in the flavour, so be sure to source it from a reputable fishmonger.

2 bunches (about 8 cups/2 L) of black dinosaur kale, tough ribs removed and sliced into ribbons

¼ cup (60 mL) extra-virgin olive oil, divided

3 tablespoons (45 mL) fresh lemon juice, divided

1 teaspoon (5 mL) sea salt

1 small fennel bulb, long fronds and top stalks trimmed off and thinly sliced

½ cup (125 mL) raw hazelnuts

5 ounces (140 g) smoked trout, flaked into bite-size pieces

1 watermelon radish, thinly sliced

1 large avocado, peeled, pitted, and diced

¼ cup (60 mL) crumbled goat cheese (optional)

Freshly ground black pepper, to taste

1. Place the kale ribbons in a large salad bowl. Add 3 tablespoons (45 mL) of the olive oil, 2 tablespoons (30 mL) of the lemon juice, and the salt. Using your hands, massage the kale for 2 to 3 minutes until it starts to soften and darken in colour. This will help tenderize the kale, making it easier to digest. Add the fennel and stir to combine.

2. Heat a dry, large skillet over medium-high heat. Add the hazelnuts in a single layer and toast, tossing occasionally, cutting board to cool. Roughly chop into pieces.

3. To serve, add the chopped hazelnuts, smoked trout, radish, avocado, and goat cheese (if using) to the salad bowl. Top with the remaining 1 tablespoon (15 mL) each of olive oil and lemon juice. Finish with some pepper.

◆ **Dairy-Free:** Skip the goat cheese.

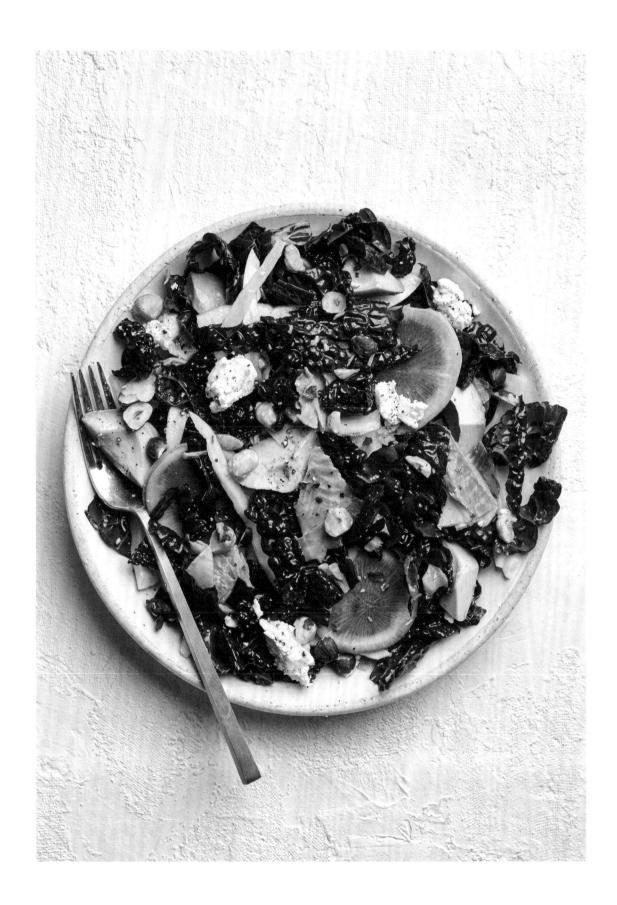

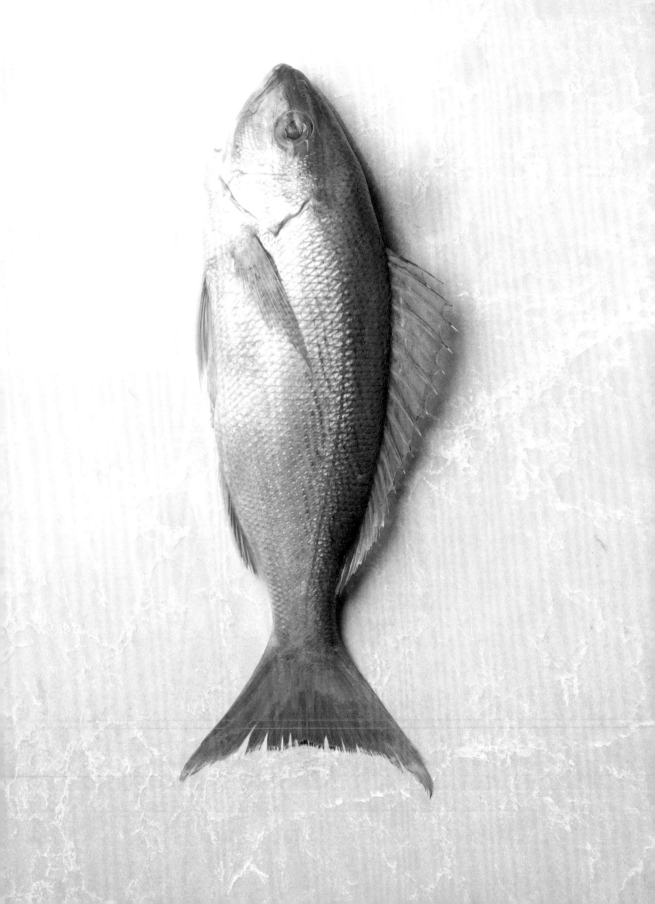

Mains
and
Sides

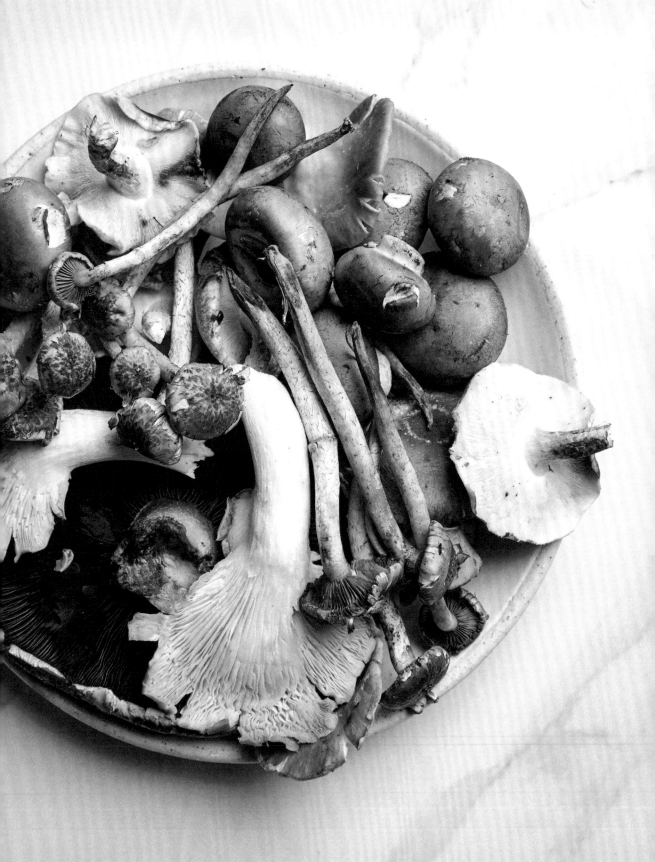

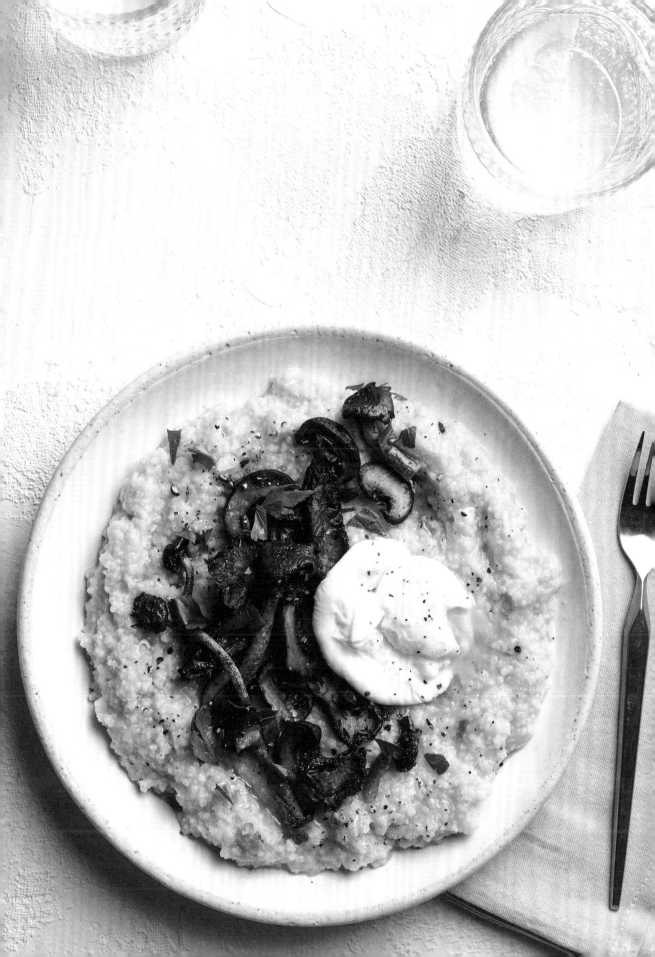

Millet Risotto with Crispy Roasted Mushrooms and a Poached Egg

This is the definition of a cozy winter meal. It has the delightful texture of millet, the cheesiness of pecorino cheese, and the butteriness of ghee. The crispy roasted mushrooms add meatiness, while the runny poached eggs add extra protein and healthy fats. This is a recipe you will want to make again and again because it is just so simple and delicious. Be sure to cook the Poached Eggs (page 268) just before serving.

Millet Risotto

1 cup (250 mL) millet

4 cups (1 L) seasoned organic chicken broth or Chicken Bone Broth (page 272), more as needed

3 tablespoons (45 mL) ghee or Plain Jane Ghee (page 271)

½ cup (125 mL) grated pecorino cheese

½ teaspoon (2 mL) sea salt

¼ teaspoon (1 mL) black pepper

Crispy Roasted Mushrooms

1 pound (450 g) assorted mushrooms (such as shiitake, oyster, and cremini)

3 tablespoons (45 mL) avocado oil

3 tablespoons (45 mL) fresh thyme leaves

1 teaspoon (5 mL) sea salt

To Serve

4 Poached Eggs (page 268)

Chopped fresh flat-leaf parsley

Extra-virgin olive oil

1. Preheat the oven to 425°F (220°C). Line a baking sheet with parchment paper.

2. **Make the Millet Risotto** Heat a dry, large skillet over medium-high heat. Add the millet in a single layer and toast, stirring occasionally, until fragrant and lightly browned, 5 to 6 minutes.

3. Transfer the millet to a food processor and pulse for 30 seconds until the grains have broken down into smaller pieces.

4. In a medium saucepan, combine the millet, chicken broth, ghee, pecorino, salt, and pepper. Bring to a boil over high heat, then reduce the heat to medium-low and simmer, covered, stirring occasionally, until the millet is tender and creamy, 25 to 30 minutes. Add ¼ to ½ cup (60 to 125 mL) more broth or water if the pot gets too dry.

5. **Meanwhile, Make the Crispy Roasted Mushrooms** Slice the mushrooms into bite-size pieces. In a medium bowl, toss the mushrooms with the avocado oil, thyme, and salt.

6. Arrange the mushrooms in a single layer on the prepared baking sheet, ensuring that there is some space between them. Roast until the mushrooms are golden brown and crispy, 25 to 30 minutes, turning them halfway through baking time.

7. To serve, divide the Millet Risotto among bowls. Top each bowl with Crispy Roasted Mushrooms, a Poached Egg, and a sprinkle of parsley. Finish with a drizzle of olive oil.

Sourdough Breaded Chicken Schnitzel with Mushroom Gravy

Schnitzel is a favourite in our household, thanks to my husband's German upbringing. Although the schnitzel is tasty all on its own, the mushroom gravy is the real star of the show. It is buttery, nutrient-dense, and delicious. This recipe calls for making homemade sourdough bread crumbs, which have a softer texture and involve freezing a loaf of sourdough bread overnight. Alternatively, you can use store-bought bread crumbs. The texture won't be quite the same, but it will still be delicious!

Mushroom Gravy

5 tablespoons (75 mL) ghee or Plain Jane Ghee (page 271), divided

1 small yellow onion, diced

1 clove garlic, minced

8 cups (2 L) sliced cremini mushrooms

Sea salt, to taste

¼ cup (60 mL) sprouted or light spelt flour (not packed)

2 cups (500 mL) seasoned organic beef broth or Beef Bone Broth (page 272)

1 tablespoon (15 mL) balsamic vinegar

½ teaspoon (2 mL) pure maple syrup

¼ teaspoon (1 mL) dried oregano

¼ teaspoon (1 mL) dried thyme

Black pepper, to taste

Sourdough Breaded Chicken Schnitzel

5 frozen slices of bread from a sourdough boule, crusts removed

4 skinless, boneless organic

chicken breasts (7½ ounces/214 g each)

1 cup (250 mL) sprouted or light spelt flour (not packed)

2 pasture-raised or organic eggs

4 to 6 tablespoons (60 to 90 mL) avocado oil, for frying

Sea salt, to taste

¼ cup (60 mL) loosely packed chopped fresh flat-leaf parsley, for garnish

Country Salad with Candied Pecans and Goat Cheese (page 93), to serve

1. **Make the Mushroom Gravy** In a large Dutch oven or a heavy-bottomed pot with a tight-fitting lid over medium-high heat, melt 2 tablespoons (30 mL) of the ghee. Add the onion and cook, stirring occasionally, until it starts to soften, 4 to 5 minutes. Add the garlic, mushrooms, and a pinch of salt. Cook, stirring often, until the liquid from the mushrooms has evaporated, 7 to 8 minutes.

2. Add the remaining 3 tablespoons (45 mL) ghee to the pot and let it melt. Add the spelt flour and stir to coat the mushrooms. Continue stirring for 2 minutes. The mixture will seem dry, but you want to toast the flour to make a roux that will help thicken the gravy.

3. Add the beef broth, balsamic vinegar, maple syrup, oregano, thyme, salt, and pepper. Bring to a boil over high heat, then reduce the heat to medium and continue cooking, stirring constantly, until the gravy has thickened, 8 to 10 minutes. Remove from the heat and cover with a lid to keep warm.

4. **Make the Sourdough Breaded Chicken Schnitzel** Cut the frozen bread into cubes and place in the bowl of a food processor fitted with the S-blade. Pulse until you have fine bread crumbs.

recipe continues

5. Place the chicken breasts on a cutting board. Working with 1 chicken breast at a time, use a meat tenderizer to pound the chicken to ½-inch (1 cm) thickness.

6. Set up a breading station by arranging 3 shallow bowls or baking dishes in a row. Add the flour to the first bowl, whisk the eggs in the second bowl, and add the bread crumbs to the third bowl. Dredge a chicken breast in the flour, shaking off any excess. Then dip the chicken breast into the egg, turning to coat it on both sides. Then carefully coat the chicken breast in the bread crumbs, pressing to ensure that they adhere to the chicken. Transfer the coated chicken breast to a baking sheet lined with parchment paper. Repeat with the remaining chicken breasts.

7. In a large cast-iron skillet over medium-high heat, heat 2 tablespoons (30 mL) of the avocado oil. Place 2 chicken breasts in the pan and cook until golden brown and crispy, 3 to 4 minutes per side. Transfer to a plate and sprinkle with salt. Wipe the crumbs from the pan and add a bit more oil before frying the remaining 2 chicken breasts. To serve, divide the chicken schnitzel among plates and top with parsley. Serve with Mushroom Gravy and Country Salad with Candied Pecans and Goat Cheese.

◆ **Dairy-Free and Nut-Free:** Skip the Country Salad with Pecans and Goat Cheese.

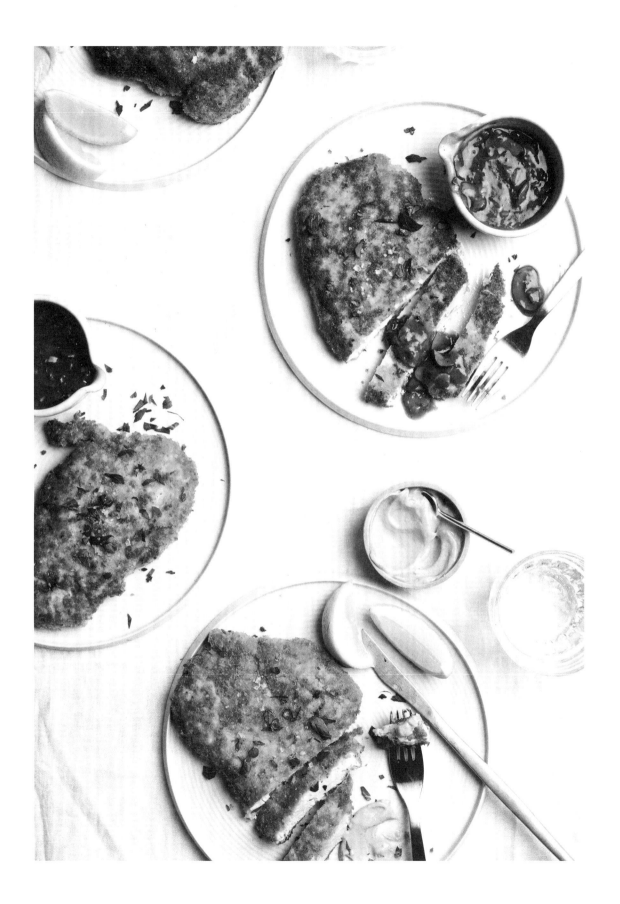

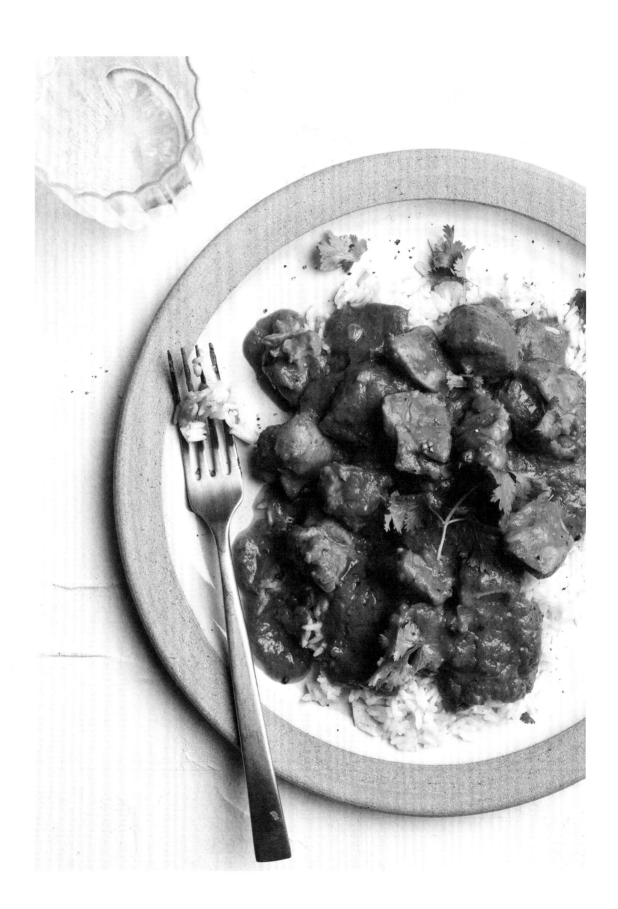

◆ Slow-Cooked Butter Chicken

My husband and I both love butter chicken, so I created this recipe that is just the way we like it—buttery and rich, with just a touch of sweetness. Chicken thighs are the fattier part of the bird, so they contain the most flavour. They are slow-cooked until they basically melt in your mouth. The best part is that this recipe is super easy to make and uses only one pot, which makes cleanup so easy. Pro tip: To make this a balanced and complete meal, add a big handful (or two) of baby spinach to the pot at the end of cooking and let it wilt.

3 tablespoons (45 mL) ghee or Plain Jane Ghee (page 271), more to serve

1 medium yellow onion, diced

2 cloves garlic, minced

1 (1-inch/2.5 cm) piece of fresh ginger, peeled and grated

1 teaspoon (5 mL) garam masala

½ teaspoon (2 mL) ground turmeric

½ teaspoon (2 mL) ground cumin

¼ teaspoon (1 mL) chili powder

¼ cup (60 mL) tomato paste

1½ cups (375 mL) canned crushed or whole tomatoes (with their juices)

2 tablespoons (30 mL) natural almond butter or Homemade Almond Butter (page 275)

⅓ cup (75 mL) canned full-fat coconut milk

½ teaspoon (2 mL) pure maple syrup

Sea salt and black pepper, to taste

2 pounds (900 g) skinless, boneless chicken thighs, cut into 1-inch (2.5 cm) pieces

To Serve

Cooked basmati rice or cauliflower rice

¼ cup (60 mL) loosely packed fresh cilantro leaves

1. In a large Dutch oven or a heavy-bottomed pot with a tight-fitting lid over medium heat, melt the ghee. Add the onion and cook, stirring occasionally, until softened, 7 to 8 minutes. Reduce the heat to low. Add the garlic, ginger, garam masala, turmeric, cumin, and chili powder. Stir to combine, then cook for 30 seconds, stirring constantly, until fragrant.

2. Add the tomato paste. Cook, stirring often, until the paste turns slightly darker in colour, 3 minutes. Add the tomatoes, almond butter, coconut milk, maple syrup, salt, and pepper. Using an immersion blender or a high-speed blender, purée the sauce until smooth.

3. Add the chicken to the saucepan with the sauce. Bring to a simmer over medium heat, then reduce the heat to medium-low. Cover and cook, stirring occasionally, for 4 hours.

4. To serve, gently stir in 1 to 2 tablespoons (15 to 30 mL) more ghee. Serve with rice and garnish with the cilantro. Store leftover butter chicken in an airtight container in the fridge for up to 7 days.

◆ **Keto-Friendly:** Skip the maple syrup. Serve with cauliflower rice.
   Paleo-Friendly: Serve with cauliflower rice.

Za'atar Roasted Chicken with Butternut Squash

My husband and I love to roast chicken together for Sunday-night dinner. This recipe came about as we were experimenting to figure out a foolproof roasting method. Since this recipe does not require trussing or turning in the oven, it is straightforward to make. The chicken has crispy ghee-roasted skin and incredibly moist meat, but the best part has to be the caramelized squash and onions soaked in the juices from the chicken. Save the bones to make Chicken Bone Broth (page 272).

¼ cup (60 mL) ghee or Plain Jane Ghee (page 271), at room temperature

3 tablespoons (45 mL) za'atar

2 teaspoons (10 mL) sea salt

1 (4-pound/1.8 kg) pasture-raised or organic chicken

3 cups (750 mL) chopped butternut squash, cut into 1-inch (2.5 cm) cubes

1 medium yellow onion, diced

6 cloves garlic, crushed

1 organic lemon

Flaky sea salt and freshly ground black pepper, to serve

1. Preheat the oven to 475°F (240°C).
2. In a small bowl, stir together the ghee, za'atar, and salt. Rub half of the ghee mixture all over the chicken, as well as under its skin. Place the chicken, breast side up, in the centre of a large cast-iron skillet.
3. In a large bowl, toss the butternut squash, onion, and garlic with the remaining ghee mixture. Arrange the squash around the chicken in a single layer. Nestle the onion and garlic between the cubes of squash.
4. Using the tip of a knife, cut slits all over the lemon. Place the lemon inside the cavity of the chicken.
5. Transfer the skillet to the oven and set a timer for 5 minutes. When the timer goes off, reduce the heat to 400°F (200°C). Roast the chicken, basting it halfway through cooking time, until the internal temperature reaches 165°F (75°C) and the juices run clear, 1 hour and 15 minutes to 1 hour and 30 minutes. Remove from the oven. Transfer the chicken to a cutting board and let it rest, uncovered, for 10 minutes.
6. Sprinkle the chicken with flaky sea salt and pepper. Carve and serve with the squash and pan juices.

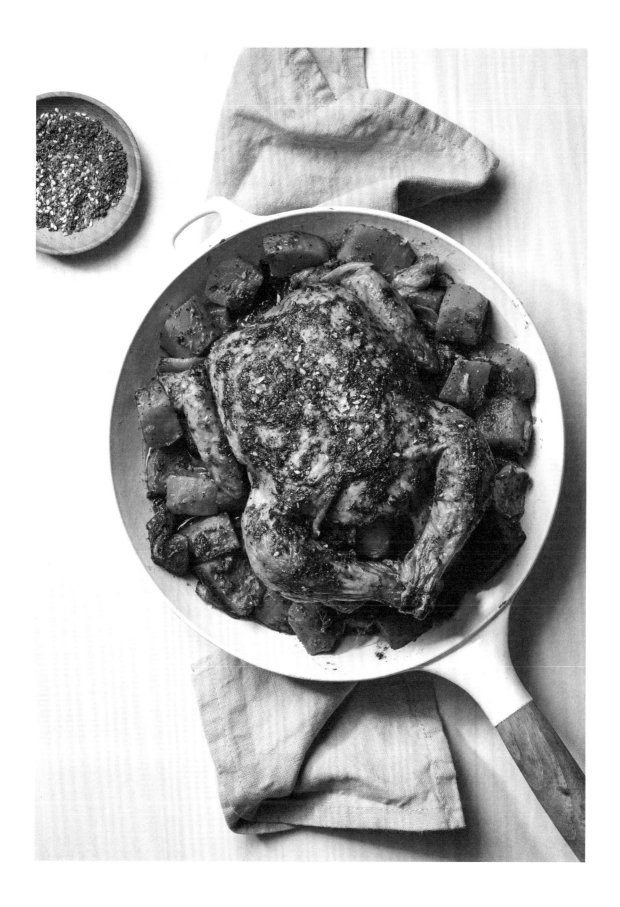

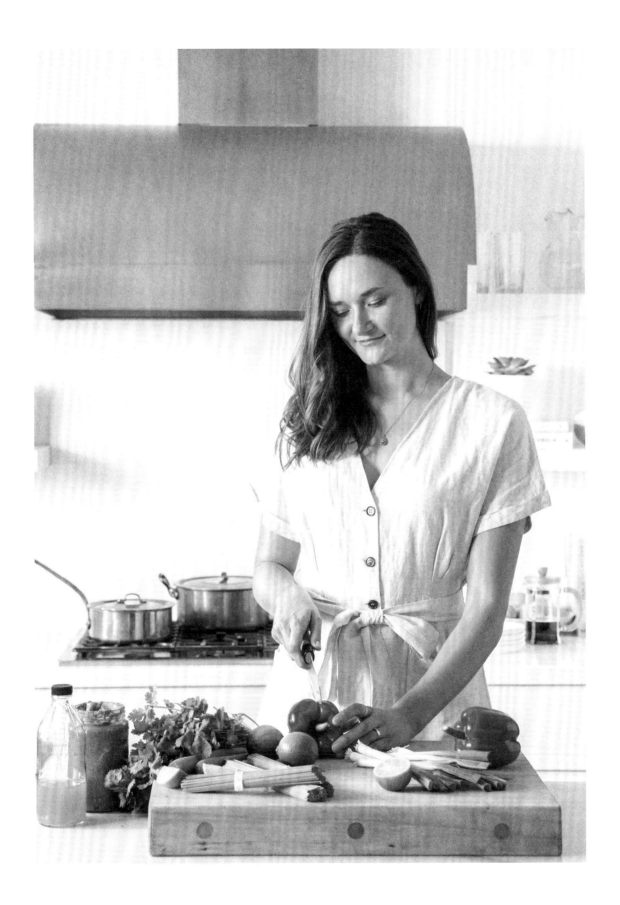

Chicken Thigh Pad Thai with Creamy Almond Butter Sauce

This is a fun variation of my favourite take-out dish. The recipe is made with organic chicken thighs instead of chicken breasts, which add a ton of flavour and good fats. The buckwheat soba noodles have a nutty flavour that complements the creamy almond butter sauce well, and they can be cooked up to 3 days ahead. In Thai dishes, it takes some time to prep all the components of the meal, but then it comes together very quickly on the stovetop. The nuts add a great crunch, so don't skimp on them.

Creamy Almond Butter Sauce

½ cup (125 mL) natural almond butter or Homemade Almond Butter (page 275)

1 tablespoon (15 mL) pure maple syrup

1 tablespoon (15 mL) gluten-free tamari

1 tablespoon (15 mL) extra-virgin olive oil

1 (1-inch/2.5 cm) piece of fresh ginger, peeled and minced

Juice from 1 lime

½ teaspoon (2 mL) sea salt

¼ cup (60 mL) water

Chicken Thigh Pad Thai

6½ ounces (185 g) gluten-free buckwheat soba noodles

1 to 2 teaspoons (5 to 10 mL) extra-virgin olive oil

2 tablespoons (30 mL) fish sauce

2 tablespoons (30 mL) apple cider vinegar

1 tablespoon (15 mL) coconut sugar

2 tablespoons (30 mL) avocado oil

5 skinless, boneless organic chicken thighs, thinly sliced (3 ounces/85 g each)

2 carrots, peeled and julienned in 2-inch (5 cm) long pieces

1 red bell pepper, seeded and thinly sliced lengthwise

1 pasture-raised or organic egg

3 green onions (white and light green parts only), thinly sliced on the diagonal

To Serve

½ cup (125 mL) chopped raw almonds or peanuts

½ cup (125 mL) loosely packed chopped fresh cilantro leaves

Lime wedges

1. **Make the Creamy Almond Butter Sauce** In a high-speed blender or a food processor, add the almond butter, maple syrup, tamari, olive oil, ginger, lime juice, salt, and water. Process on high speed for 25 to 30 seconds, until smooth.

2. **Make the Chicken Thigh Pad Thai** Fill a large saucepan halfway with unsalted water and bring to a boil over high heat. Add the soba noodles and ensure that all noodles are submerged in the water. Cook, uncovered, for exactly 3 minutes. Drain the noodles.

3. Using a fine mesh strainer, rinse the noodles thoroughly under cold running water. Transfer to a large bowl, drizzle immediately with the olive oil, and toss to coat (this will help prevent the noodles from sticking together).

4. In a small bowl, combine the fish sauce, apple cider vinegar, and coconut sugar. Stir until the coconut sugar is dissolved.

recipe continues

recipe continued

5. In a large cast-iron skillet or a wok, heat the avocado oil over high heat. Add the fish sauce mixture, chicken thighs, carrots, and bell pepper. Stir-fry, stirring occasionally, until all of the liquid is absorbed and the chicken is cooked through and golden brown, 8 to 10 minutes.

6. Reduce the heat to medium. Push the chicken and vegetables to one side of the pan. Crack the egg into the open space and roughly scramble the egg using a wooden spoon. Cook for 15 to 20 seconds, stirring constantly, until the egg is fully cooked. Mix the egg, chicken, and vegetables together, stirring to combine.

7. Add the noodles, green onions, and all of the Creamy Almond Butter Sauce. Using tongs, toss everything well to combine. Cook for 2 to 3 minutes, until the noodles are reheated.

8. To serve, divide the Chicken Thigh Pad Thai among plates or shallow bowls. Garnish with the chopped almonds and cilantro. Serve with lime wedges.

Pan Seared Grass-Fed Steaks with Crispy Roasted Potatoes

Grass-fed steaks are a good source of omega-3 fatty acids and protein to enjoy occasionally as part of a healthy diet. Pan searing steaks in ghee is an excellent choice because of its high smoke point and rich, buttery flavour. All you need is a side of roasted asparagus and a salad and you have an easy and impressive dinner. Pro tip: You can season the steaks with salt and pepper as soon as you get them home from the store (up to 2 days ahead of cooking). This will help the seasonings penetrate deeper into the meat.

Pan Seared Grass-Fed Steaks

6 grass-fed top sirloin steaks (each 6 ounces/170 g and about 1¼-inches/3 cm thick)

Sea salt and black pepper, to taste

2 tablespoons (30 mL) Ghee, Plain Jane Ghee (page 271) or duck fat, for searing

Flaky sea salt, to serve

Crispy Roasted Potatoes

6 organic Yukon Gold potatoes, peeled and quartered

6 cloves garlic, peeled

¼ cup (60 mL) melted ghee, Plain Jane Ghee (page 271), or duck fat

2 tablespoons (30 mL) fresh thyme leaves, roughly chopped

2 tablespoons (30 mL) fresh oregano leaves, roughly chopped

Sea salt and black pepper, to taste

Flaky sea salt, to serve

Avocado Rocket Salad with Mustard Lemon Vinaigrette (page 101), to serve

1. Position two racks in the upper and lower thirds of the oven. Preheat the oven to 375°F (190°C). Pat the steaks dry and season generously with salt and pepper. Let sit at room temperature while you make the Crispy Roasted Potatoes.

2. **Make the Crispy Roasted Potatoes** Fill a large saucepan halfway with salted water and bring to a boil over high heat. Add the potatoes and boil, uncovered, for 10 minutes, until softened around the edges but still very firm on the inside.

3. Drain the potatoes thoroughly and add them to a large bowl. Shake the bowl to fluff up the edges of the potatoes (this will help make them crispy). Add the garlic, ghee, thyme, oregano, salt, and pepper. Toss to coat. Transfer to a baking sheet, spreading the potatoes evenly in a single layer, flat sides down. Roast on the upper rack until the outside of the potatoes are golden brown and crispy, 50 to 60 minutes, turning the potatoes halfway through baking time. Remove the potatoes from the oven and immediately sprinkle them with flaky sea salt. Leave the oven set at 375°F (190°C) to cook the steaks.

4. **Pan-Sear the Grass-Fed Steaks** Turn on the exhaust fan (and open the windows!). In a 12-inch (30 cm) cast-iron skillet over high heat, heat 1 tablespoon (15 mL) of ghee. Lay the steaks in the pan (they will fit snugly but shrink as they cook). Sear for 2 to 3 minutes until a crust forms on the bottom. Add another tablespoon (15 mL) of ghee to the pan and flip the steaks. Sear for 2 minutes on the other side.

recipe continues

recipe continued

5. Transfer the pan to the lower rack in the oven and cook for 4 to 6 minutes for medium-rare doneness, 8 to 10 minutes for medium doneness, or 12 to 14 minutes for medium-well doneness. Remove from the oven and transfer the steaks to a cutting board. Let rest for 10 to 15 minutes. Turn off the oven and place the potatoes in the oven to stay warm.

6. Slice the steaks and transfer them to a platter. Top with the pan juices and sprinkle with flaky sea salt. Serve with Crispy Roasted Potatoes and Avocado Rocket Salad with Mustard Lemon Vinaigrette (page 101).

◆   **Dairy-Free:** Skip the cheese in the Avocado Rocket Salad.
    Nut-Free: Skip the nuts in the Avocado Rocket Salad.

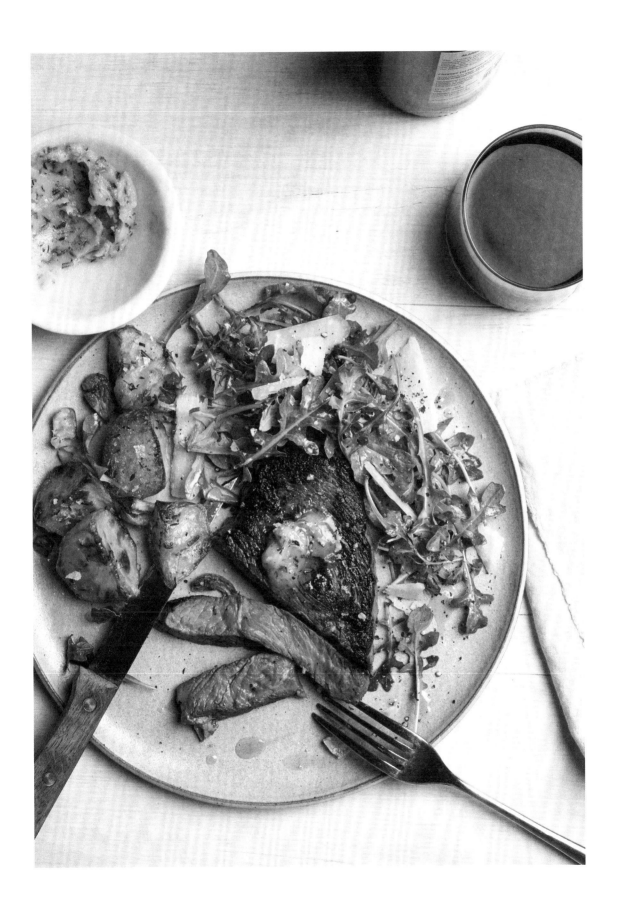

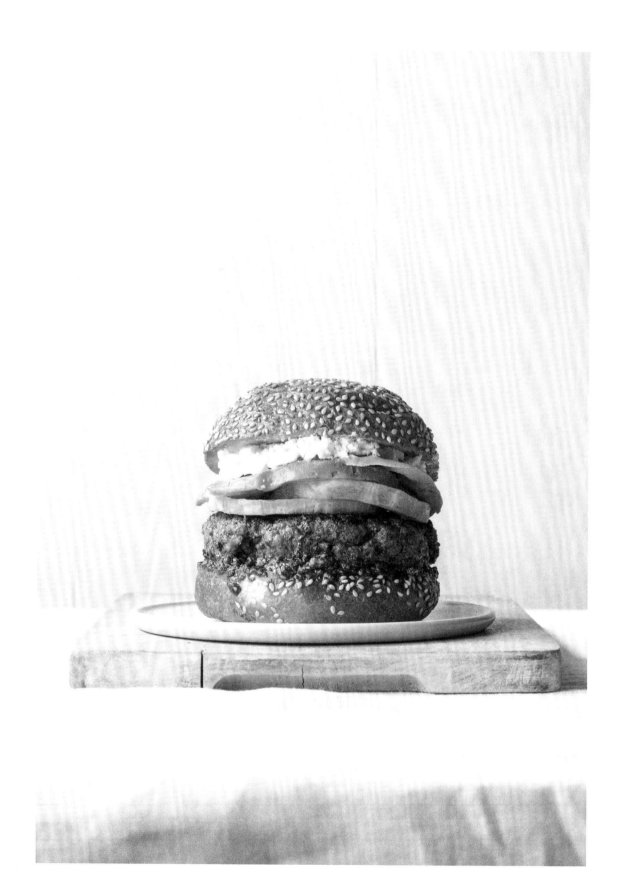

Grass-Fed Burgers with Pesto and Butternut Squash

Burgers are generally not considered healthy, but when you make them from grass-fed beef, they are an excellent source of omega-3 fatty acids and protein. Cooking the burgers in ghee makes them buttery and irresistible. You can save on preparation time by roasting the butternut squash ahead and using store-bought pesto instead of making it from scratch. The burgers are delicious served on brioche buns, but they can also be served on a bed of lettuce.

1 small butternut squash, peeled, halved, and seeded

1 tablespoon (15 mL) avocado oil

Sea salt and black pepper, to taste

1½ pounds (675 g) grass-fed ground beef

1 tablespoon (15 mL) melted ghee or Plain Jane Ghee (page 271), for brushing the pan

4 brioche buns or gluten-free buns, sliced in half

To Serve

Pesto or Fresh Pesto (page 276)

Sliced avocado

Crumbled goat cheese (optional)

1. Preheat the oven to 400°F (200°C).
2. Cut the butternut squash into ¼-inch (5 mm) slices. In a large bowl, toss the squash with the avocado oil, salt, and pepper. Arrange in a single layer on a baking sheet. Roast until fork-tender, 20 to 25 minutes.
3. Divide the ground beef into 4 equal portions. Roll each portion into a ball, then flatten with the palm of your hand to form ¾-inch (2 cm) thick patties. Season generously with salt and pepper on both sides.
4. Heat a large cast-iron skillet over medium-high heat. Add the ghee and reduce the heat to medium-high. Place the patties in the pan and cook, undisturbed, for 4 minutes. Flip and cook for 4 to 5 more minutes (4 minutes for medium-rare doneness, 5 minutes for medium doneness). Remove the burgers from the pan.
5. In the same pan (no need to wipe the pan), add 2 buns, cut side down. Toast until golden brown on the bottom, about 30 seconds. Repeat with the remaining 2 buns.
6. To serve, spread the pesto on the bottom half of each bun and add the patties. Top with a slice or two of roasted butternut squash, along with sliced avocado and goat cheese, if using.

◆ **Gluten-Free:** Serve the burgers on gluten-free buns.
Grain-Free: Serve the burgers on a bed of butter lettuce instead of on buns.
Keto-Friendly: Serve the burgers on a bed of butter lettuce instead of on buns. Skip the butternut squash.

◆ Healthyish Carbonara

This carbonara recipe is a grown-up version of my mother's bacon, egg, and cheese pasta I ate as a child. The secret to good carbonara is using high-quality, organic, pasture-raised eggs (the ones with the bright orange yolks). The egg yolks act as the sauce, lending nutrients as well as plenty of good fats. I love to use quinoa spaghetti, as it does not get mushy when it is cooked, unlike some of the other gluten-free spaghetti varieties.

12 ounces (340 g) quinoa or chickpea spaghetti

4 ounces (115 g) organic bacon, cut into small pieces

1 pasture-raised or organic egg

6 pasture-raised or organic egg yolks

⅓ cup (75 mL) grated pecorino cheese, more to serve

¾ teaspoon (4 mL) freshly ground black pepper, more to serve

1. In a large saucepan, bring 4 quarts (4 L) of salted water to a boil. Once the water is boiling, add the spaghetti. Cook according to the package directions, until al dente. Drain the pasta, reserving 2 tablespoons (30 mL) of the cooking water.

2. Meanwhile, cook the bacon. In a medium skillet over medium heat, cook the bacon, flipping it every 2 to 3 minutes until crispy on both sides, 8 to 10 minutes. Remove from the heat.

3. In a large bowl, whisk together the egg and egg yolks. Add the bacon along with its rendered fat, pecorino, pepper, and the reserved cooking water. Whisk to combine. Add the pasta to the bowl. Using tongs, toss the pasta to coat it in the egg mixture.

4. To serve, divide the carbonara among plates. Serve with additional grated pecorino and black pepper.

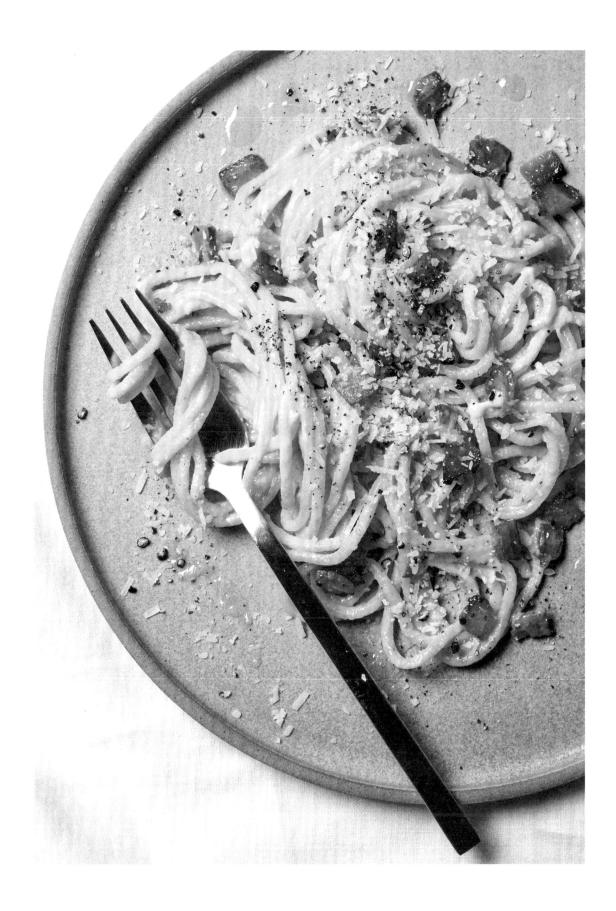

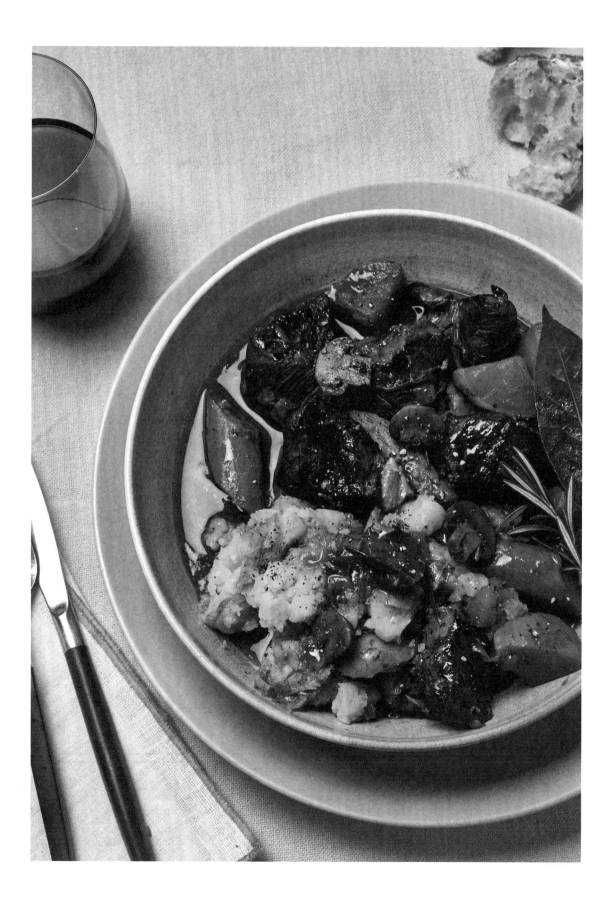

◆ Braised Lamb Stew with Root Vegetables

If you like lamb as much as I do, then you will love this braised lamb stew. Pasture-raised lamb has plenty of good fats, including conjugated linoleic acid (CLA) and omega-3 fatty acids. Plus, most lamb comes from Australia and New Zealand, where it is pasture-raised, so you can buy it at a regular grocery store without having to worry. I suggest serving this stew over mashed parsnips or with some crusty sourdough bread for a hearty, satisfying meal that will hug you from the inside out.

2 pounds (900 g) boneless, pasture-raised leg of lamb, cut into 1½-inch (4 cm) cubes

Sea salt and black pepper, to taste

2 tablespoons (30 mL) ghee or Plain Jane Ghee (page 271), more as needed

1 large yellow onion, diced

2 tablespoons (30 mL) tomato paste

1 cup (250 mL) dry red wine

2 teaspoons (10 mL) arrowroot starch

4 cups (1 L) seasoned organic beef broth or Beef Bone Broth (page 272), divided

8 ounces (225 g) button mushrooms, sliced in half (about 2½ cups/625 mL)

5 medium carrots, peeled and sliced on the diagonal into 1½-inch (4 cm) pieces (about 2½ cups/625 mL)

2 small turnips, peeled and cut into 1½-inch (4 cm) cubes (about 2 cups/500 mL)

2 bay leaves

1 head of garlic, halved crosswise

2 sprigs of fresh rosemary

1. Preheat the oven to 350°F (180°C).
2. Pat the lamb dry and season with salt and pepper on all sides. In a large Dutch oven or a heavy-bottomed pot with a tight-fitting lid over medium-high heat, melt the ghee. Working in batches and being careful not to overcrowd the pan, brown the lamb for 2 to 3 minutes per side. Add more ghee as needed. Set the browned lamb aside while you prepare the base of the stew.
3. Reduce the heat to medium. Add the onion and cook, stirring occasionally, until just softened, about 2 minutes. Add the tomato paste and cook, stirring constantly, for 1 minute. Add the wine and stir to deglaze the pan. Bring to a simmer over medium heat and cook for 4 to 5 minutes, stirring occasionally, until slightly thickened.
4. In a small bowl, whisk the arrowroot starch with 2 tablespoons (30 mL) of the beef broth until smooth. Add to the pot and stir to combine. Add the remaining broth, browned lamb with the juices, mushrooms, carrots, turnips, bay leaves, garlic, and rosemary. Submerge the vegetables in the liquid and bring to a boil over high heat. Cover the pot, place in the oven, and cook until the lamb is tender, about 2 hours. Season with salt and pepper. Discard the garlic halves, rosemary stems, and bay leaves.
5. To serve, ladle the stew into bowls.

Moroccan Lamb Meatballs with Yogurt-Tahini Sauce

These juicy Moroccan meatballs are baked in the oven for a hassle-free cleanup. I use a combination of ground lamb and grass-fed ground beef, which makes them really moist and delicious. The Yogurt-Tahini Sauce, crumbled feta, and olive oil add a healthy dose of fats and creaminess, while the vibrant garnishes of olives, tomato, and cucumber add freshness and make for a beautiful presentation.

Moroccan Lamb Meatballs

1 pound (450 g) pasture-raised ground lamb

1 pound (450 g) grass-fed ground beef

½ cup (125 mL) panko or gluten-free bread crumbs

¼ cup (60 mL) loosely packed chopped fresh mint leaves

1 tablespoon (15 mL) ground cumin

2 teaspoons (10 mL) sweet paprika

2 teaspoons (10 mL) sea salt

½ teaspoon (2 mL) cayenne pepper

½ teaspoon (2 mL) ground ginger

½ teaspoon (2 mL) ground cinnamon

½ teaspoon (2 mL) black pepper

1 medium red onion, coarsely grated

Yogurt-Tahini Sauce

1 cup (250 mL) plain full-fat yogurt

⅓ cup (75 mL) tahini

¼ cup (60 mL) loosely packed fresh mint leaves

2 cloves garlic

½ teaspoon (2 mL) sea salt

To Serve

1 tablespoon (15 mL) extra-virgin olive oil

Pinch of Aleppo pepper or red chili flakes

¼ cup (60 mL) pitted Kalamata olives

Sliced Persian or English cucumber

1 large heirloom tomato, sliced into wedges

Crumbled sheep's or goat's milk feta cheese (optional)

1. Preheat the oven to 425°F (220°C). Line a baking sheet with parchment paper.
2. **Make the Moroccan Lamb Meatballs** In a large bowl, add all of the ingredients for the meatballs. Using your hands, mix together the ingredients. Scoop the mixture into ¼ cup (60 mL) portions and form them into balls.
3. Arrange the meatballs on the prepared baking sheet. Bake until the internal temperature reaches 165°F (74°C) or until the meatballs are browned and cooked through, 18 to 20 minutes.
4. **Meanwhile, Make the Yogurt-Tahini Sauce** In a high-speed blender or a food processor, combine the yogurt, tahini, mint, garlic, and salt. Blend on high speed until smooth, 10 to 15 seconds. Depending on the thickness of the yogurt and tahini, you may need to add a bit of water to thin the sauce to desired consistency.
5. To serve, pour the Yogurt-Tahini Sauce onto plates. Drizzle with the olive oil and sprinkle with Aleppo pepper. Place the meatballs on top of the sauce. Serve with kalamata olives, cucumber, tomato wedges, and crumbled feta, if using.

◆ **Dairy-Free:** Use coconut yogurt instead of dairy yogurt. Skip the feta cheese.
Gluten-Free: Use gluten-free bread crumbs instead of panko.

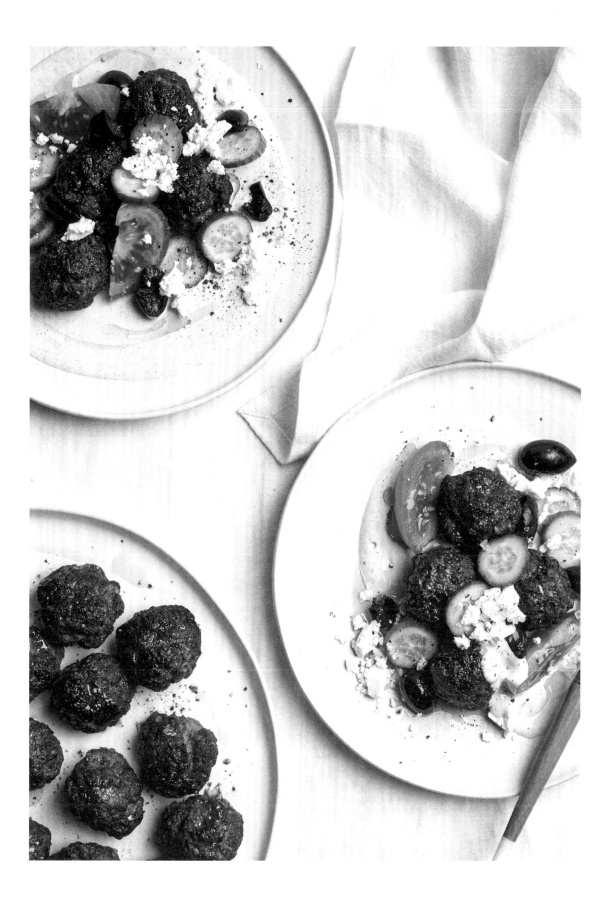

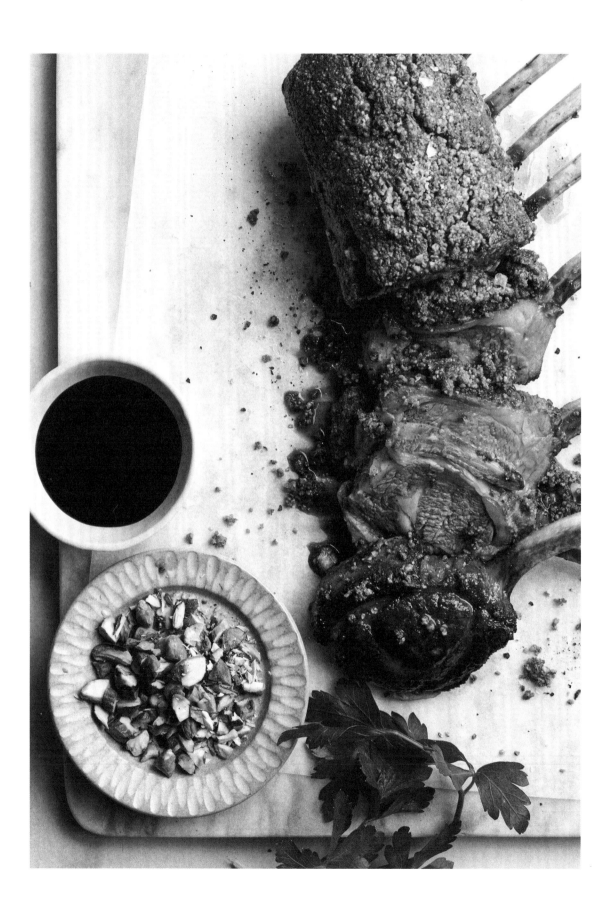

Pistachio-Crusted Rack of Lamb with Pomegranate Butter Glaze

This recipe was a massive hit with our recipe testers, and I am not surprised given how delicious it is! Pomegranate molasses is the perfect balance of tart and sweet, and the pistachio crust adds a lovely texture. The main thing to note is that since rack of lamb is such a precious cut, take extra care not to overcook it. If your oven is on the hot side, you'll want to err on the side of caution and check for doneness after 15 minutes. You will need to remove the lamb from the fridge 1 hour before cooking to bring it to room temperature. This ensures that the meat stays tender in the oven.

Pistachio-Crusted Rack of Lamb

1 pasture-raised rack of lamb (about 1½ pounds/675 g), frenched

Sea salt and black pepper, to taste

½ cup (125 mL) raw shelled pistachios

2 tablespoons (30 mL) panko or gluten-free bread crumbs

¼ cup (60 mL) loosely packed chopped fresh flat-leaf parsley

1 tablespoon (15 mL) ghee or Plain Jane Ghee (page 271), at room temperature

¼ teaspoon (1 mL) sea salt

1 tablespoon (15 mL) avocado oil

Pomegranate Butter Glaze

2 tablespoons (30 mL) pomegranate molasses

2 teaspoons (10 mL) ghee or Plain Jane Ghee (page 271), at room temperature

¼ teaspoon (1 mL) garlic powder

Pinch of cinnamon

Pinch of ground cumin

Pinch of sweet paprika

1. Position a rack in the lower third of the oven. Preheat the oven to 350°F (180°C). Line a baking sheet with foil.
2. **Make the Pistachio-Crusted Rack of Lamb** Using a sharp knife, slice off the thick layer of fat on top of the rack of lamb. Season generously with salt and pepper on all sides.
3. In a food processor, combine the pistachios, bread crumbs, parsley, ghee, and salt. Pulse until ground into a coarse meal.
4. In a large cast-iron skillet over high heat, heat the avocado oil. Place the lamb in the pan and brown, 2 to 3 minutes per side. Transfer to the prepared baking sheet, bone side down.
5. **Make the Pomegranate Butter Glaze** In a small bowl, combine the pomegranate molasses, ghee, garlic powder, cinnamon, cumin, and paprika. Spread the glaze over the top side of the lamb. Press the pistachio mixture onto the glaze in a thick, even layer.
6. Bake for 15 to 20 minutes for rare doneness or 20 to 25 minutes for medium-rare doneness. Transfer the lamb to a cutting board and let it rest for 10 minutes. Using a sharp knife, carefully carve between each set of bones. Serve immediately.

◆ **Gluten-Free:** Use gluten-free bread crumbs instead of panko.

Sheet Pan Sausage Dinner with Caramelized Cabbage and Red Onion

This is one of my favourite dinners when I want something simple and delicious. It has the right balance of sweet, salty, spicy, and acidic flavours that makes each bite irresistible. Although oven-baked sausages are always delightful, the wedges of caramelized cabbage and red onion cooked in the juices are the real stars of the show. If you want a bit of extra spiciness, use hot Italian sausages instead of mild ones—just be sure to source your sausages from a reputable butcher shop or farmers market. This is a dish you will want to make again and again!

½ small green cabbage, tough outer leaves removed

1 red onion, peeled and halved

6 cloves garlic

¼ cup (60 mL) melted ghee or Plain Jane Ghee (page 271)

1 tablespoon + 1½ teaspoons (22 mL) pure maple syrup

1 teaspoon (5 mL) red chili flakes

Sea salt and black pepper, to taste

5 organic mild Italian sausages (18 ounces/500 g total)

4 sprigs of fresh rosemary

2 tablespoons (30 mL) apple cider vinegar

1 tablespoon (15 mL) extra-virgin olive oil

Flaky sea salt and freshly ground black pepper, to serve

1. Position a rack in the middle of the oven. Preheat the oven to 425°F (220°C).

2. Slice the cabbage and red onion into 1-inch (2.5 cm) thick wedges. Place the wedges on an unlined baking sheet, then add the garlic cloves.

3. In a small bowl, whisk together the melted ghee, maple syrup, chili flakes, salt, and pepper.

4. Drizzle the ghee mixture over the vegetables and gently toss to coat, keeping each wedge intact as much as possible. Arrange the vegetables in an even layer, leaving space between each wedge.

5. Prick the sausages with a knife a few times on each side. Place the sausages and rosemary sprigs over the vegetables. Roast until the sausages are cooked through and golden brown on top, 45 minutes to 1 hour. The vegetables should be golden brown and caramelized around the edges when ready.

6. To serve, transfer the sausages and vegetables to a serving platter. Drizzle with the apple cider vinegar and olive oil. Sprinkle with flaky sea salt and pepper.

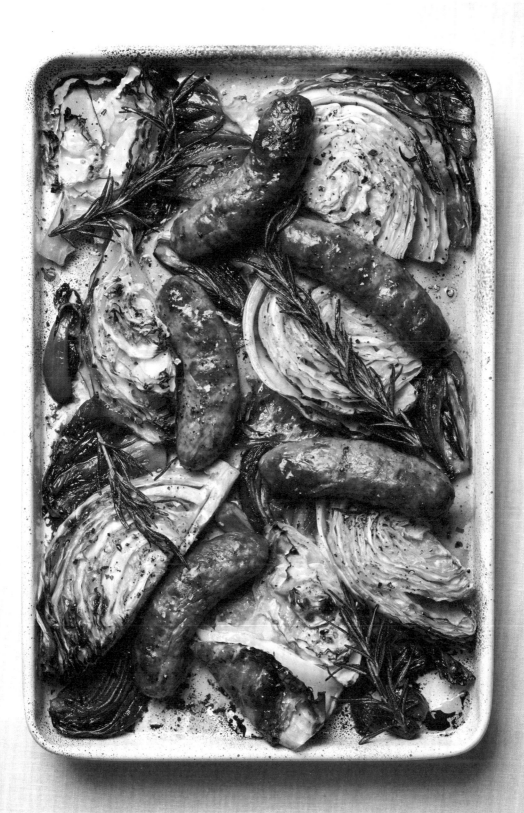

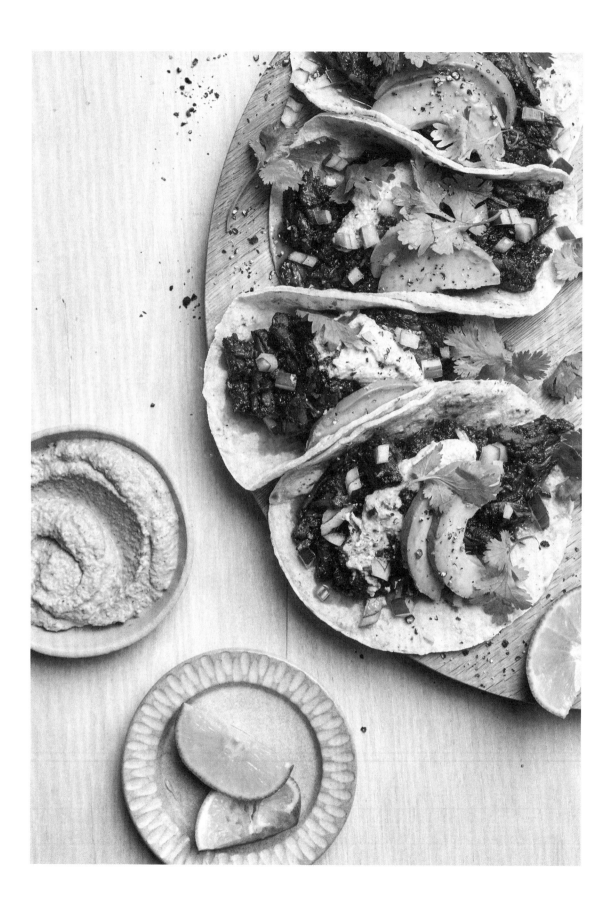

Beef Barbacoa Tacos

This barbacoa taco filling is made with grass-fed brisket, which is slow-cooked with Mexican spices until it becomes melt-in-your-mouth tender. Grass-fed brisket can be found at well-stocked grocery stores and some butcher shops. The slow cooking in step 3 can also be done in an Instant Pot (1 hour on high pressure) and yield the same results. This recipe makes a generous amount of barbacoa filling—any leftover meat can be used to top grain bowls and salads throughout the week.

Adobo Sauce

2 cloves garlic

1 chipotle pepper in adobo sauce

1 small yellow onion, diced

2 tablespoons (30 mL) fresh lime juice

1 tablespoon (15 mL) apple cider vinegar

1½ teaspoons (7 mL) ground cumin

1½ teaspoons (7 mL) dried oregano

½ cup (125 mL) seasoned organic beef broth or Beef Bone Broth (page 272)

1 teaspoon (5 mL) sea salt

½ teaspoon (2 mL) black pepper

Beef Barbacoa

2 pounds (900 g) grass-fed beef brisket, fat trimmed and cut into 2-inch (5 cm) cubes

Sea salt and black pepper, to taste

2 tablespoons (30 mL) avocado oil, more as needed

2 bay leaves

Cilantro-Lime Cashew Crema

¾ cup (175 mL) raw cashews, soaked in room-temperature water for at least 8 hours, drained, and rinsed

½ cup (125 mL) packed chopped fresh cilantro leaves and stems

1 jalapeño pepper, seeded

3 tablespoons (45 mL) fresh lime juice

2 cloves garlic, roughly chopped

¾ teaspoon (4 mL) sea salt

½ cup (125 mL) water

To Serve

12 soft corn tortillas

2 avocados, peeled, pitted, and sliced

½ cup (125 mL) loosely packed fresh cilantro leaves

Diced red onion

Fresh lime wedges

1. **Make the Adobo Sauce** In a high-speed blender or a food processor, add the garlic, chipotle pepper, onion, lime juice, apple cider vinegar, cumin, oregano, beef broth, salt, and pepper. Blend on high speed until smooth, 10 to 15 seconds.

2. **Make the Beef Barbacoa** Pat the meat dry and season with salt and pepper on all sides. In a large Dutch oven or a heavy-bottomed pot with a tight-fitting lid over medium-high heat, heat the avocado oil. Working in small batches and being careful not to overcrowd the pot, brown the beef for 2 to 3 minutes on each side. Add more oil as needed.

3. Add the Adobo Sauce and bay leaves to the pot. Reduce the heat to medium-low. Simmer, covered, until the beef is very tender, 3 to 4 hours.

4. Remove the bay leaves and transfer the beef to a large bowl. Using 2 forks, shred the beef. Return the beef to the pot and cover to keep warm.

recipe continues

recipe continued

5. **Make the Cilantro-Lime Cashew Crema** In a high-speed blender or a food processor, combine the soaked cashews, cilantro, jalapeño, lime juice, garlic, salt, and water. Blend on high speed until smooth, 20 to 30 seconds.

6. Heat a large skillet over medium-high heat. Working in batches, add 2 or 3 tortillas to the pan and warm them for 30 seconds per side.

7. To serve, divide the Beef Barbacoa among the tortillas. Top with Cilantro-Lime Cashew Crema, sliced avocado, cilantro, and red onion. Serve with lime wedges.

◆ **Grain-Free and Paleo-Friendly:** Use leaves of butter lettuce instead of corn tortillas.
Nut-Free: Skip the Cilantro-Lime Cashew Crema.

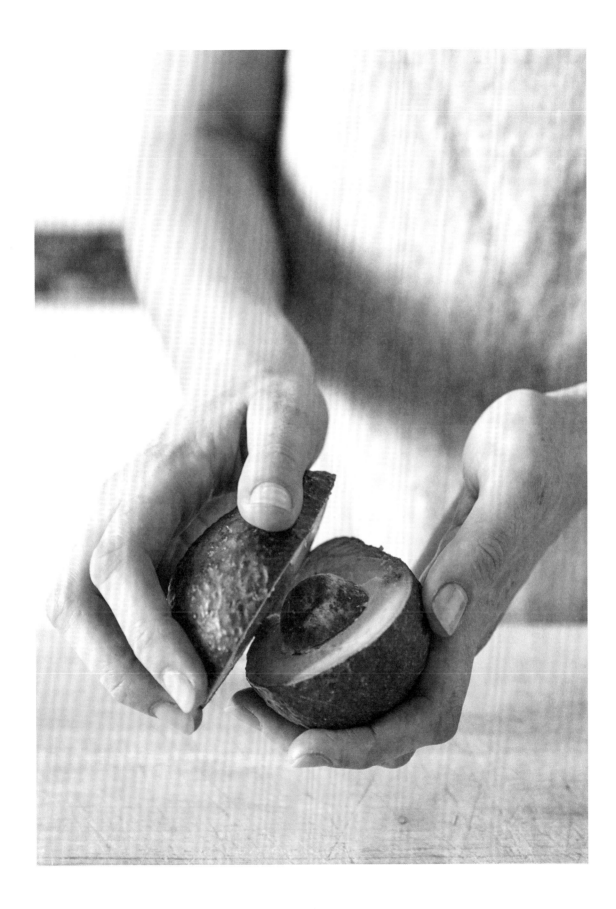

◆ Crispy Beer Battered Fish Tacos

Fish tacos are one of my greatest pleasures in life. When my favourite local taco joint shut down, I was forced to learn how to make these tacos at home. They are made with sustainably caught Icelandic cod, which is an excellent source of heart-healthy omega-3 fatty acids. To fry the cod, I use avocado oil for its high smoke point and neutral flavour. These tacos share the same toppings as the Beef Barbacoa Tacos (page 143). I suggest making both recipes and serving them for a taco party!

2 pounds (900 g) wild-caught Icelandic cod, skinned and filleted

1 cup (250 mL) sprouted or light spelt flour or 1:1 gluten-free all-purpose flour, divided (not packed)

1½ teaspoons (7 mL) arrowroot starch

¾ teaspoon (4 mL) sea salt, more to taste

1 cup (250 mL) lager beer, such as Modelo, or gluten-free beer

Avocado oil, for frying

To Serve

12 soft corn tortillas

Cilantro-Lime Cashew Crema (page 143)

2 avocados, peeled, pitted, and sliced

½ cup (125 mL) loosely packed fresh cilantro leaves

Diced red onion

Fresh lime wedges

Hot sauce, such as Cholula (optional)

1. Cut the cod lengthwise into strips about 3-inches (8 cm) long and 1-inch (2.5 cm) wide. Pat the strips dry.

2. In a shallow baking dish, add ¼ cup (60 mL) of the spelt flour. Add the cod strips and toss to coat.

3. In a medium bowl, combine the remaining ¾ cup (175 mL) spelt flour, arrowroot starch, and salt. Add the beer, whisking to combine. The batter should have the consistency of pancake batter. If the batter is too thin, whisk in a bit more flour. If the batter is too thick, add another splash of beer and whisk to combine.

4. Place a rack on top of a baking sheet. This will be used later for the fried fish, to keep it crispy and drain off excess oil.

5. In a large cast-iron skillet or a Dutch oven, add a ⅛-inch (3 mm) layer of avocado oil. Heat the oil over medium-high heat. Test the temperature by placing a drop of batter in the pan. If it sizzles immediately and floats to the top, the oil is hot enough.

6. Working in batches, coat 5 or 6 pieces of fish, one at a time, in the batter. Let excess batter drip back into the bowl and place the coated fish in the pan, ensuring that they don't touch each other. Fry until the batter is golden brown and crisp, 2 to 3 minutes per side. Add more oil as needed. Using tongs or a metal fish spatula, remove the fish from the pan and place it on the prepared rack. Sprinkle with salt. Repeat with the remaining fish, then wipe the pan clean.

7. Reduce the heat to medium. In the same pan, working in batches, add 2 or 3 tortillas and warm them for 30 seconds to 1 minute per side. Repeat with the remaining tortillas.

8. To serve, divide the fish among the tortillas. Top with Cilantro-Lime Cashew Crema, sliced avocado, cilantro, and red onion. Serve with lime wedges and hot sauce, if using.

◆ **Gluten-Free:** Use gluten-free all-purpose flour instead of sprouted or light spelt flour. Use gluten-free beer.

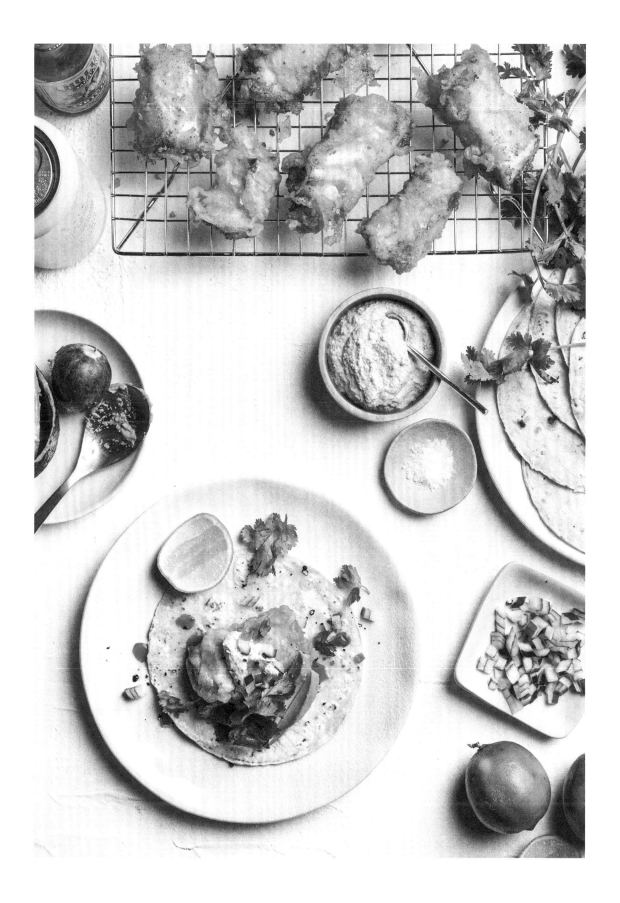

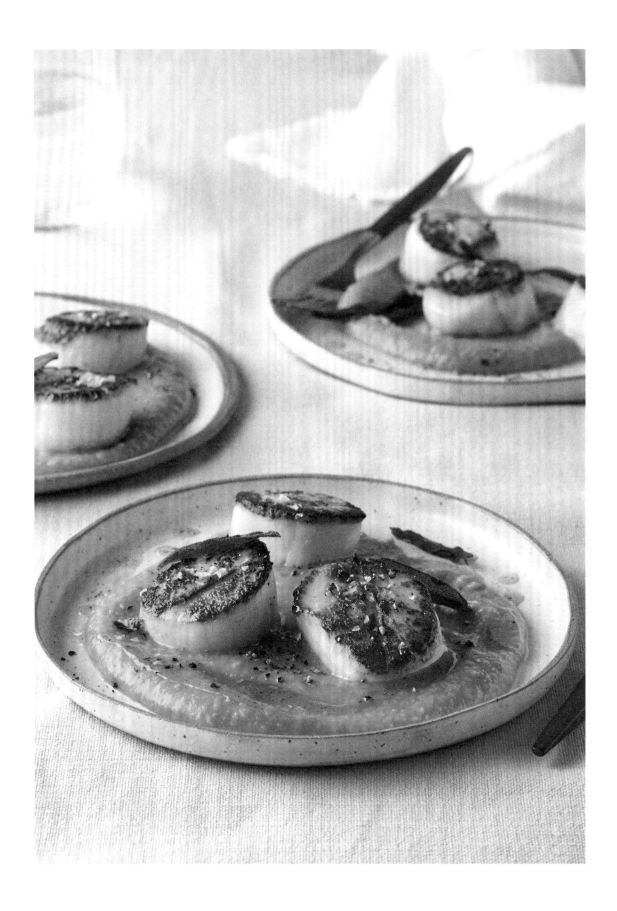

Seared Scallops with Crispy Sage and Kabocha Squash Purée

Scallops are one of the healthiest seafood choices, because they are low in mercury and high in omega-3 fats, including EPA and DHA, which are essential for brain health. A lot of people are intimidated by scallops, but this foolproof recipe shows how simple they are to make. I sear the scallops in ghee for its high smoke point and buttery flavour, but if you can get your hands on some brown butter ghee, it takes this dish to a whole new level. I serve these scallops with a side of roasted asparagus or broccolini. Kabocha squash is only in season from late summer to early fall. If you can't find it, use buttercup squash instead. Save the leftover squash to make a batch of Kabocha Squash Cupcakes with Dulce de Coco (page 241) for dessert!

Kabocha Squash Purée

1 small kabocha or buttercup squash (about 2 pounds/900 g), cut in half and seeded

3 tablespoons (45 mL) avocado oil, divided

1 small yellow onion, minced

2 cloves garlic, minced

1 cup (250 mL) seasoned organic vegetable broth

⅓ cup (75 mL) canned full-fat coconut milk

1 teaspoon (5 mL) sea salt

Seared Scallops with Crispy Sage

12 colossal sea scallops

½ teaspoon (2 mL) sea salt

3 tablespoons (45 mL) ghee, Plain Jane Ghee (page 271), or brown butter ghee

¼ cup (60 mL) loosely packed fresh sage leaves

Flaky sea salt and freshly ground black pepper, to serve

1. Preheat the oven to 400°F (200°C). Line a baking sheet with parchment paper.
2. **Make the Kabocha Squash Purée** In a large bowl, coat the squash with 1 tablespoon (15 mL) of the avocado oil, then place it, cut side down, on the prepared baking sheet. Roast until the squash is fork-tender, 30 to 35 minutes. Scoop out the flesh of half the squash and put it in a high-speed blender or a food processor.
3. In a medium skillet over medium heat, heat the remaining 2 tablespoons (30 mL) avocado oil. Add the onion and garlic and cook, stirring occasionally, until softened, 5 to 7 minutes. Add the vegetable broth, coconut milk, and salt and bring to a simmer over medium-high heat. Remove from the heat and carefully add the mixture to the blender or food processor. Blend on high speed to form a smooth purée, 15 to 20 seconds. Cover to keep warm.
4. **Make the Seared Scallops with Crispy Sage** Pat the scallops dry and season with the salt on all sides.
5. In a large cast-iron skillet over medium-high heat, melt the ghee. Add the scallops, leaving space between each one. Cook, undisturbed, until dark golden brown, 2 to 3 minutes per side. Transfer the scallops to a plate.
6. Add the sage leaves to the pan. Cook until the sage leaves are crisp and dark green around the edges, 5 to 10 seconds.
7. To serve, divide the Kabocha Squash Purée among plates. Top with the seared scallops and crispy sage leaves. Spoon the ghee from the pan over the scallops, then sprinkle with flaky sea salt and pepper.

Masala Roasted Branzino with Turmeric Cashew Rice

My friend Rory, an avid cook, suggested I come up with a whole fish recipe to go with my favourite turmeric rice recipe. This fish is full of flavour from the masala spice blend, and the turmeric cashew rice is a vibrant side dish that complements the fish perfectly. Don't be intimidated by the idea of cooking a fish whole—it is much easier than you think and makes for a beautiful main course!

Turmeric Cashew Rice

1 cup (250 mL) long-grain brown rice

2 cups (500 mL) seasoned organic vegetable broth

3 tablespoons (45 mL) ghee or Plain Jane Ghee (page 271)

1 small yellow onion, diced

1 cup (250 mL) raw cashews

1½ teaspoons (7 mL) ground turmeric

1 teaspoon (5 mL) ground cumin

1 teaspoon (5 mL) sea salt

5 green Thai chilies, thinly sliced (optional)

Masala Roasted Branzino

2 whole branzino (3 pounds/ 1.35 kg total), scaled and gutted

1 to 2 teaspoons (5 to 10 mL) avocado oil

2 teaspoons (10 mL) garam masala

Sea salt and black pepper, to taste

1 organic lemon, thinly sliced

¼ cup (60 mL) loosely packed fresh cilantro leaves, for garnish

1. Preheat the oven to 425°F (220°C). Line a baking sheet with parchment paper.

2. **Make the Turmeric Cashew Rice** In a medium pot, combine the rice with the vegetable broth and bring to a boil. Reduce to a simmer, cover, and cook until the rice is tender, 35 to 40 minutes. Remove from the heat and fluff with a fork. Cover to keep warm.

3. In a medium skillet over medium-high heat, melt the ghee. Add the onion and cook, stirring often, until soft and translucent, 5 to 7 minutes. Add the cashews, turmeric, cumin, and salt. Cook, stirring occasionally, until the cashews are lightly toasted and golden brown, 2 to 3 minutes. Add the cashew mixture and green chilies (if using) to the rice and stir to combine. Cover to keep warm while you roast the branzino.

4. **Make the Masala Roasted Branzino** Pat the fish dry, inside and out. Brush the outside of the fish with the avocado oil. Sprinkle the garam masala, salt, and pepper on both sides of each fish.

5. Place a few lemon slices inside each fish. Place the fish on the prepared baking sheet and roast until the flesh flakes easily with a fork, 14 to 18 minutes. Be careful not to overcook the fish.

6. You can either serve the fish whole or fillet the fish. To fillet each fish, place it on a cutting board. Using a sharp knife, cut off the head and tail. Make a slit along the top edge of the fish. Using a flat spatula, carefully lift the top fish fillet away from the spine, leaving the skin intact. Holding the fish by the tail end, lift the spine of the fish away from the bottom fillet and discard. Check carefully to ensure that no bones remain in the fish. Repeat to fillet the second fish. You will have 2 fillets from each fish, 4 in total.

7. Serve the fish with Turmeric Cashew Rice and garnish with the cilantro.

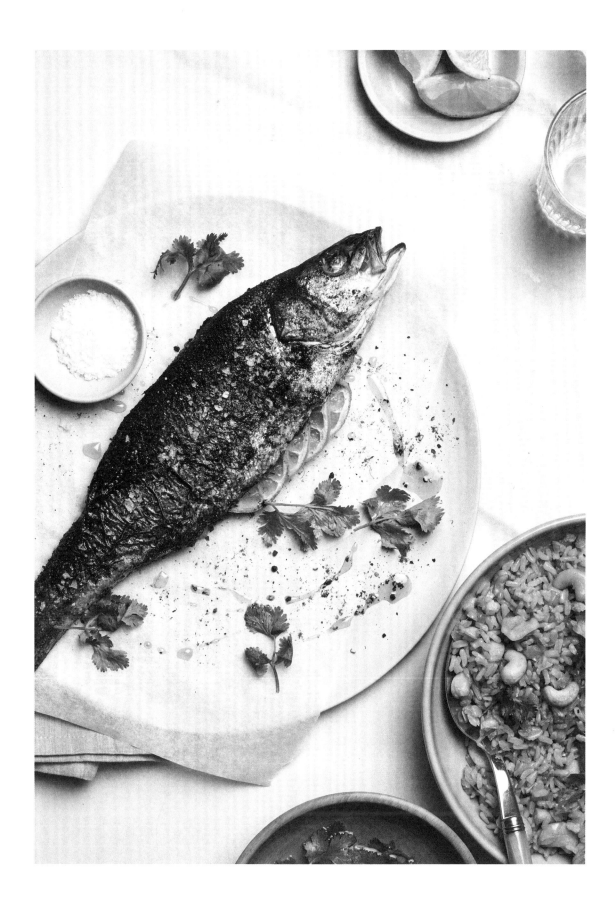

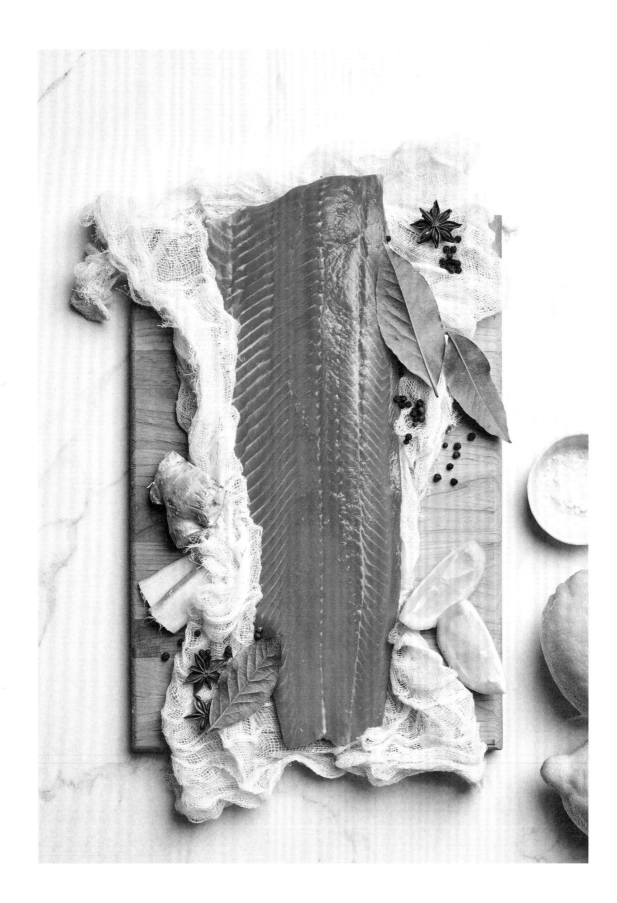

Poached Steelhead Trout with Lemon Aioli

Poaching fish, which gently cooks fish in a flavourful liquid, is a technique I learned from my grandmother's family recipe book. Poaching ensures that the fish does not dry out and highlights its delicate texture. Although it may seem tedious to cook the vegetables individually, this is necessary due to their various cooking times. Steelhead trout is a close relative of salmon that is full of healthy omega-3 fatty acids.

6 cups (1.5 L) water

1 tablespoon + 1½ teaspoons (22 mL) sea salt

1 (2-inch/5 cm) piece of fresh ginger, peeled and grated

6 black peppercorns, crushed

1 star anise

3 bay leaves

1 pound (450 g) baby potatoes, cut in half

8 young carrots with tops, peeled, halved lengthwise, and tops trimmed to ½ inch (1 cm)

12 ounces (340 g) asparagus or green beans, ends trimmed

½ cup (125 mL) dry white wine

1¼ pounds (565 g) skin-on steelhead trout fillet

3 tablespoons (45 mL) ghee or Plain Jane Ghee (page 271), at room temperature, divided

To Serve

Flaky sea salt, to taste

Lemon Aioli (page 277) or fresh lemon wedges

1. In a large, oval-shaped Dutch oven or a heavy-bottomed pot with a tight-fitting lid, bring the water to a boil. Add the salt, ginger, peppercorns, star anise, and bay leaves. Reduce the heat to medium and simmer, covered, for 5 to 6 minutes to create a flavourful poaching liquid.

2. Add the potatoes and carrots and bring the liquid back to a boil over medium-high heat. Cover and boil the vegetables until fork-tender, 6 to 8 minutes. Using tongs, remove the vegetables from the boiling water and transfer them to a colander.

3. Add the asparagus to the pot and let the liquid come back to a boil. Cover and blanch the asparagus until crisp-tender. Using tongs, remove the asparagus from the boiling water and transfer it to the colander with the potatoes and carrots.

4. Add the wine to the pot. Reduce to a simmer over medium heat.

5. Place the trout, skin side up, on 2 layers of 3-foot (90 cm) long cheesecloth. Holding the ends of the cheesecloth, carefully lower the fish into the poaching liquid, ensuring that the thickest part is fully submerged. Leave the ends of the cheesecloth draped over the sides of the pot, cover, and then fold the cheesecloth over the lid. Poach the fish until it flakes easily with a fork, 5 to 7 minutes. Carefully lift the fish out of the liquid and transfer it to a serving platter. Discard the cheesecloth. Dot the flesh of the trout with 1 tablespoon (15 mL) of the ghee and sprinkle with flaky sea salt.

6. In a large skillet over medium-high heat, melt the remaining 2 tablespoons (30 mL) ghee. Add the vegetables to the skillet and gently toss to coat them in ghee. Reheat the vegetables for 1 to 2 minutes. Arrange them on another serving platter and sprinkle with flaky sea salt.

7. To serve, carefully flake the trout into 4 pieces, separating the flesh from the skin. Discard the skin. Serve with Lemon Aioli or fresh lemon wedges.

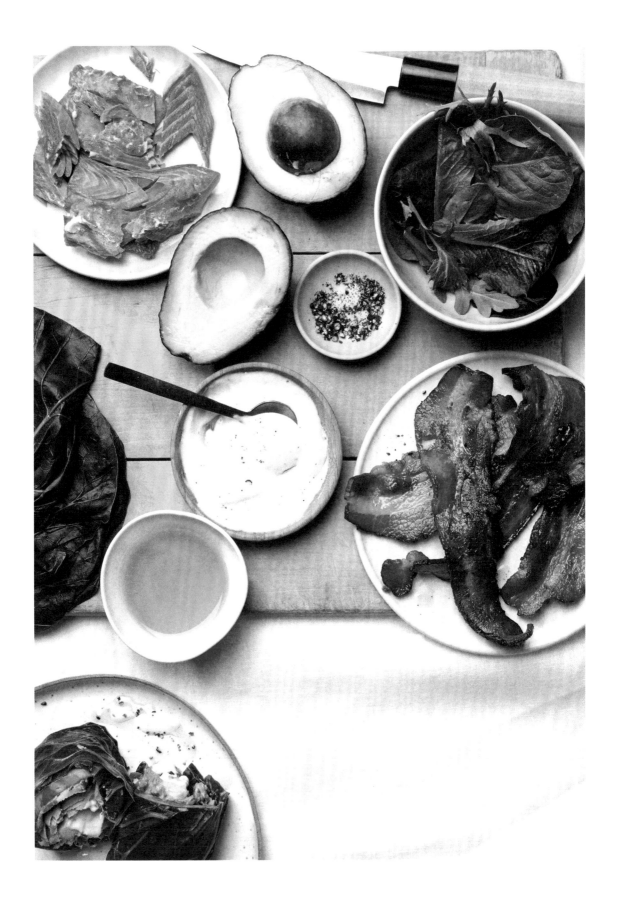

Dairy-Free ◆ Gluten-Free Option ◆ Grain-Free Option ◆ Nut-Free
◆ Keto-Friendly Option ◆ Paleo-Friendly Option ◆ *Serves 2*

Salmon Avocado Club Wraps

I make this club wrap when I have leftover Lemon Aioli (page 277) and Perfect Oven Bacon (page 270). You should use a bit less filling than you think you need, so as not to overstuff the wrap and have it tear and fall apart. Whole-grain wraps can be found at well-stocked grocery stores; just make sure to get the largest ones you can find. For a lighter option, you can also use steamed collard wraps. Don't throw away the crispy salmon skin—it is delicious!

5 ounces (140 g) skin-on wild salmon fillet

Sea salt and black pepper, to taste

1 tablespoon (15 mL) avocado oil

2 large whole-grain wraps or collard wraps (see Grain-Free Option)

Lemon Aioli (page 277) or mayonnaise

4 slices of Perfect Oven Bacon (page 270), cut into bite-size pieces

Sliced avocado

Sliced tomato

Spring mix

1. Position a rack in the middle of the oven. Preheat the oven to 200°F (100°C).

2. Season the salmon on both sides with salt and pepper. In a large cast-iron skillet over medium-high heat, heat the avocado oil. Add the salmon fillet, skin side down. Reduce the heat to medium and cook, undisturbed, until the skin is crispy, 3 to 5 minutes. Flip and cook for another 2 to 3 minutes, until the salmon is cooked all the way through. Transfer the salmon to a cutting board. Using a fork, flake the salmon into bite-size pieces.

3. Place the wraps directly on the rack in the oven and heat until warm, 1 to 2 minutes.

4. Spread some Lemon Aioli onto each wrap. Pile the flaked salmon, bacon pieces, avocado, tomato, and spring mix in the centre of each wrap, leaving 2 inches (5 cm) of space on the top, bottom, and sides.

5. Working with one wrap at a time, fold in the sides until they are nearly touching. Roll up the bottom of the wrap over the filling, squeezing the filling to secure the shape. Continue rolling until the entire wrap is rolled up. Slice in half.

◆ **Gluten-Free:** Use gluten-free wraps instead of whole-grain wraps.
 Grain-Free, Keto-Friendly, and Paleo-Friendly: Use collard wraps instead of whole-grain wraps. Blanch 2 large collard leaves in boiling water until they soften and turn vibrant green, about 1 minute. Transfer the collard leaves to a bowl of ice water, then drain. Slice off the tough part of the stem and fill and wrap as described above.

Miso-Orange Wild Salmon with Black Rice and Crispy Broccolini

This is an uncomplicated, all-in-one dinner that is simple enough to make on a weeknight yet impressive enough for a dinner party with friends. Wild-caught salmon is full of omega-3 fatty acids, which are great for your memory and cardiovascular health. The delicately flavoured salmon looks beautiful on a bed of black rice. Warning: The crispy broccolini is highly addictive, so you may want to make a double batch.

Miso-Orange Wild Salmon

1 cup (250 mL) pure orange juice

¼ cup (60 mL) white miso paste

2 tablespoons (30 mL) pure maple syrup

1 teaspoon (5 mL) garlic powder

4 skin-on wild salmon fillets (6 ounces/170 g each)

Sea salt and black pepper, to taste

2 tablespoons (30 mL) avocado oil

Black Rice

2 cups (500 mL) seasoned organic vegetable broth

1 cup (250 mL) short-grain black forbidden rice

1 teaspoon (5 mL) ghee or Plain Jane Ghee (page 271)

¼ teaspoon (1 mL) sea salt

Crispy Broccolini

1 bunch of broccolini, 1 inch (2.5 cm) cut off ends

2 tablespoons (30 mL) avocado oil

¼ teaspoon (1 mL) sea salt

¼ teaspoon (1 mL) black pepper

¼ teaspoon (1 mL) garlic powder

Pinch of cayenne pepper

To Serve

1 tablespoon (15 mL) gluten-free tamari

1 teaspoon (5 mL) toasted sesame oil

1 tablespoon (15 mL) sesame seeds

1. Preheat the oven to 400°F (200°C).

2. **Make the Miso-Orange Marinade** In a small bowl, whisk together the orange juice, miso paste, maple syrup, and garlic powder.

3. Place the salmon fillets, skin side down, in a small baking dish. Pour the marinade over top. Cover with a clean kitchen towel and marinate in the fridge for 30 to 45 minutes.

4. **Meanwhile, Cook the Black Rice** In a medium saucepan, bring the vegetable broth to a boil. Add the black rice, ghee, and salt. Reduce the heat to medium-low and cook until the rice is soft and chewy, 35 to 40 minutes.

5. **Meanwhile, Make the Crispy Broccolini** Slice any thick broccolini pieces in half or into thirds lengthwise so that all pieces are about the same thickness.

6. In a large bowl, toss the broccolini with the avocado oil, salt, pepper, garlic powder, and cayenne. Arrange the broccolini in a single layer on an unlined baking sheet, leaving some space between each piece. Roast until crispy, 15 to 20 minutes.

recipe continues

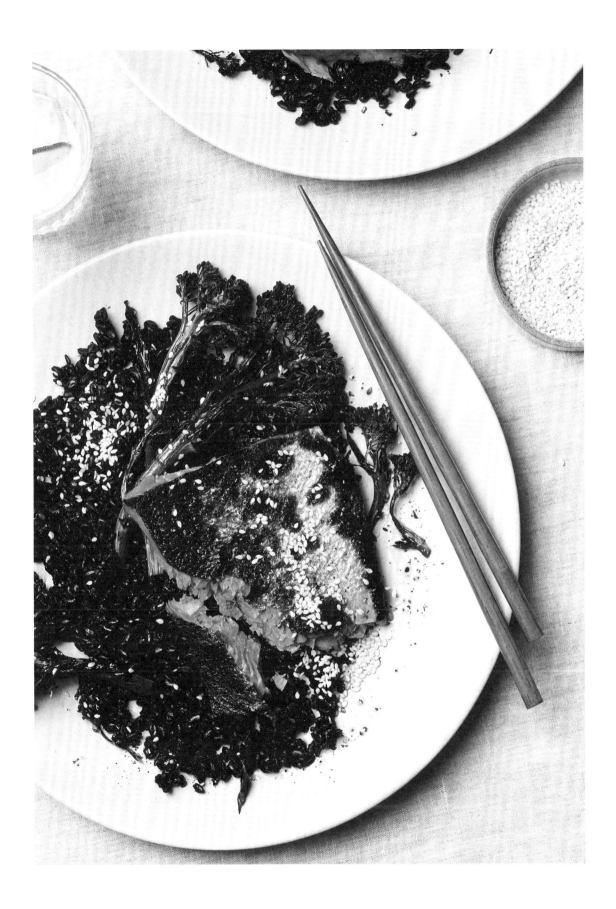

recipe continued

7. **Sear the Salmon** Remove the salmon from the marinade and discard the marinade. Season the salmon on both sides with salt and pepper. In a large skillet over medium-high heat, heat the avocado oil. Place the salmon fillets, skin side down, in the pan. Reduce the heat to medium and cook, undisturbed, until the skin is crispy, 3 to 5 minutes. Flip and cook for another 2 to 3 minutes, until the salmon is cooked all the way through.

8. To serve, divide the rice among plates. Place the crispy broccolini and seared salmon over top. Drizzle with the tamari and toasted sesame oil, then sprinkle with the sesame seeds.

Salmon Avocado Poke Bowl with Sweet Potato Tempura Bites

This fresh, energizing bowl has fibre, protein, good fats, and complex carbohydrates—which means it will keep you full for hours on end. Smoked salmon and avocado are both excellent sources of heart-healthy fats. The sweet potato tempura bites are made with a gluten-free tempura batter that gets really crispy when fried in avocado oil. Usually, poke bowls use sushi-grade tuna, but I use smoked salmon because it is lower in mercury and higher in omega-3 fatty acids.

Salmon Avocado Poke Bowl

3 cups (750 mL) water

1½ cups (375 mL) short-grain brown rice, rinsed and drained

1 tablespoon (15 mL) ghee or Plain Jane Ghee (page 271)

2 sheets of nori, cut into 1-inch (2.5 cm) long strips

5 ounces (140 g) smoked sockeye salmon, chopped into bite-size pieces

1 red bell pepper, diced

1 cup (250 mL) diced English cucumber

2 avocados, peeled, pitted, and sliced

2 green onions (white and light green parts only), thinly sliced

½ cup (125 mL) thinly sliced purple cabbage

2 tablespoons (30 mL) sesame seeds

Sweet Potato Tempura Bites

½ cup (125 mL) arrowroot starch

¼ cup (60 mL) coconut flour

1 teaspoon (5 mL) baking powder

1 teaspoon (5 mL) sea salt, more to taste

½ cup (125 mL) water

1 pasture-raised or organic egg

Avocado oil, for frying

1 small sweet potato, peeled, quartered lengthwise, and cut into ¼-inch (5 mm) thick slices

Tamari Dressing

¼ cup (60 mL) extra-virgin olive oil

¼ cup (60 mL) gluten-free tamari

¼ cup (60 mL) apple cider vinegar

1 tablespoon (15 mL) pure maple syrup

½ teaspoon (2 mL) garlic powder

1. **Cook the Brown Rice** In a medium saucepan, bring the water to a boil. Add the rice and ghee. Reduce to a simmer and cook, covered, until the rice is tender, 45 to 50 minutes.

2. **Meanwhile, Make the Sweet Potato Tempura Bites** In a medium bowl, whisk together the arrowroot starch, coconut flour, baking powder, salt, water, and egg. The batter should be smooth.

3. Place a rack on top of a baking sheet. This will be used later for the fried tempura bites, to keep them crispy and drain off excess oil.

4. In a large cast-iron skillet or a Dutch oven, add a ⅛-inch (3 mm) layer of avocado oil. Heat the oil over medium-high heat. Test the temperature by placing a drop of batter in the pan. If it sizzles immediately and floats to the top, the oil is hot enough.

recipe continues

5. Working in batches of 10 to 12 pieces, dip the sweet potato slices, one at a time, in the batter. Let excess batter drip back into the bowl and place the coated slices in the pan, ensuring that they don't touch each other. Fry until the batter is golden brown and crisp, 1 to 2 minutes per side. Add more oil as needed. Using tongs or a metal fish spatula, remove the tempura bites from the pan and place them on the prepared rack. Sprinkle with salt. Repeat with the remaining sweet potato slices. Discard the leftover oil and batter.

6. **Make the Tamari Dressing** In a small bowl, whisk together the olive oil, tamari, apple cider vinegar, maple syrup, and garlic powder.

7. To serve, divide the rice among bowls and top with Sweet Potato Tempura Bites, nori strips, smoked salmon, bell pepper, cucumber, avocado, green onion, and cabbage. Drizzle each bowl with Tamari Dressing and sprinkle with the sesame seeds.

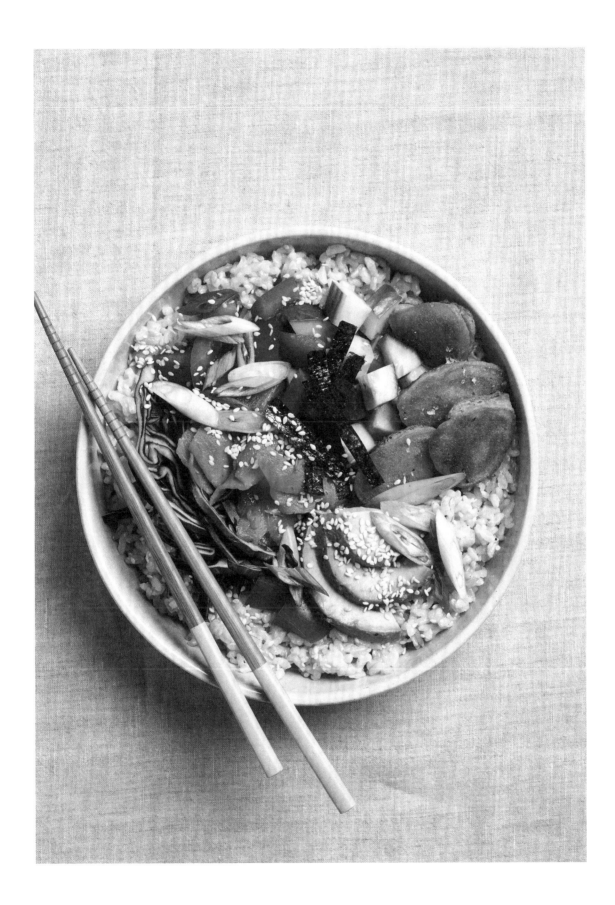

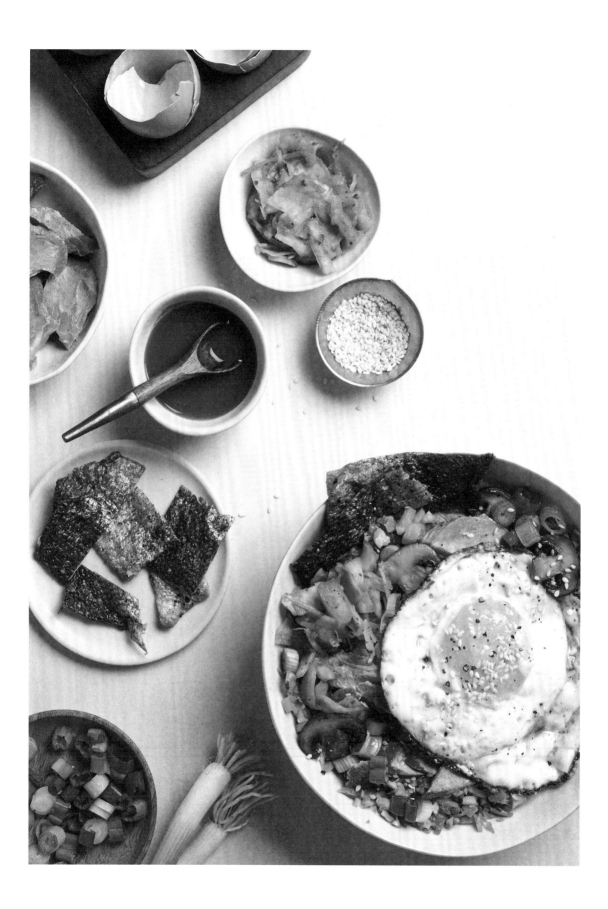

Dairy-Free ◆ Gluten-Free ◆ Grain-Free ◆ Nut-Free
◆ Keto-Friendly Option ◆ Paleo-Friendly Option ◆ *Serves 4*

Brassica Bibimbap Bowls with Wild Salmon

I eat wild salmon every chance I can, and this bowl is such a delicious way to get more salmon into your diet. It is full of flavour and has three different vegetables from the brassica family: broccoli, cauliflower, and fermented cabbage (kimchi). It also has plenty of protein and healthy fats from salmon, sesame seeds, and eggs. These days, you can find riced cauliflower and riced broccoli at well-stocked grocery stores, which makes life a whole lot easier. Cook the Ghee-Fried Eggs (page 269) just before serving.

5 tablespoons (75 mL) avocado oil or ghee, divided

4 cups (1 L) sliced cremini mushrooms

Sea salt, to taste

3 cups (750 mL) riced broccoli

3 cups (750 mL) riced cauliflower

1 (1-inch/2.5 cm) piece of fresh ginger, peeled and minced

2 cloves garlic, minced

3 tablespoons (45 mL) gluten-free tamari or coconut aminos

8 ounces (225 g) skin-on wild salmon fillet

Black pepper, to taste

To Serve

4 Ghee-Fried Eggs (page 269)

½ cup (125 mL) chopped kimchi

¼ cup (60 mL) sliced green onion (white and light green parts only)

Toasted sesame oil

2 tablespoons (30 mL) sesame seeds

Hot sauce (optional)

1. In a large skillet over medium-high heat, heat 2 tablespoons (30 mL) of the avocado oil. Add the mushrooms and cook, stirring often, until golden and crispy, 2 to 3 minutes. Transfer the mushrooms to a small bowl and sprinkle them with salt.

2. Add 2 tablespoons (30 mL) avocado oil to the pan. Add the riced broccoli, riced cauliflower, ginger, garlic, and tamari. Sauté over medium-high heat, stirring often, until the vegetables are tender, 7 to 8 minutes. Transfer the brassica mixture to a medium bowl and wipe the pan clean.

3. Season the salmon on both sides with salt and pepper. In the same pan over medium-high heat, heat the remaining 1 tablespoon (15 mL) avocado oil. Place the salmon, skin side down, in the pan. Reduce the heat to medium and cook, undisturbed, until the skin is crispy, 3 to 5 minutes. Flip and cook for another 2 to 3 minutes, until the salmon is cooked all the way through.

4. Transfer the salmon to a cutting board. Using a fork, flake the salmon into bite-size pieces. Chop the crispy salmon skin.

5. To serve, divide the brassica mixture among bowls. Top each bowl with mushrooms, flaked salmon, crispy salmon skin, Ghee-Fried Eggs, kimchi, and green onion. Drizzle with toasted sesame oil and garnish with the sesame seeds. Serve with hot sauce, if desired.

◆ **Keto-Friendly and Paleo-Friendly**: Use coconut aminos instead of gluten-free tamari.

Rainbow Pesto Grain Bowls

This is a healthy and satisfying grain bowl. The flavour of the pesto tossed with the rainbow of vegetables really takes it to the next level. Although various steps are involved, you can make the vegetables, pesto, and grains ahead to have them ready for easy lunches during the week. I love the array of colours in this recipe, but feel free to use whichever vegetables you happen to have on hand.

3 tablespoons (45 mL) ghee or Plain Jane Ghee (page 271), at room temperature

1 teaspoon (5 mL) ground turmeric

1 small head of cauliflower, cut into large bite-size pieces

1 small head of red cabbage, quartered, one quarter cut into 4 wedges, core intact

2 tablespoons (30 mL) avocado oil, divided

Sea salt and black pepper, to taste

1 red bell pepper, seeded and cut into 8 sections

1 zucchini, ends trimmed and sliced on the diagonal into ¾-inch (2 cm) thick slices

1 small sweet potato, peeled and diced into ¾-inch (2 cm) cubes

To Serve

3 cups (750 mL) cooked brown rice, millet, or quinoa

½ cup (125 mL) pesto or Fresh Pesto (page 276)

4 Ghee-Fried Eggs (page 269)

1. Position racks in the upper and lower thirds of the oven. Preheat the oven to 450°F (230°C). Line 2 baking sheets with parchment paper.

2. In a large bowl, combine the ghee and turmeric. Add the cauliflower and, using your hands, massage the ghee all over it. Arrange in a single layer on one side of a prepared baking sheet.

3. Place the 4 cabbage wedges in a single layer on the other side of the baking sheet. Drizzle 1½ teaspoons (7 mL) of the avocado oil on one side of the cabbage wedges, then season with a bit of salt and pepper. Turn the wedges over and drizzle 1½ teaspoons (7 mL) avocado oil over the other side, then season with a bit more salt and pepper.

4. In a large bowl, toss the bell pepper, zucchini, and sweet potato with the remaining 1 tablespoon (15 mL) avocado oil, salt, and pepper. Arrange the vegetables in a single layer on the second prepared baking sheet.

5. Roast both sheets of vegetables until tender and golden brown, 25 to 30 minutes, turning the vegetables and switching the sheets on the racks halfway through the baking time.

6. To serve, divide the cooked grains among 4 large bowls. Top each with a large spoonful of pesto, roasted vegetables, and a Ghee-Fried Egg.

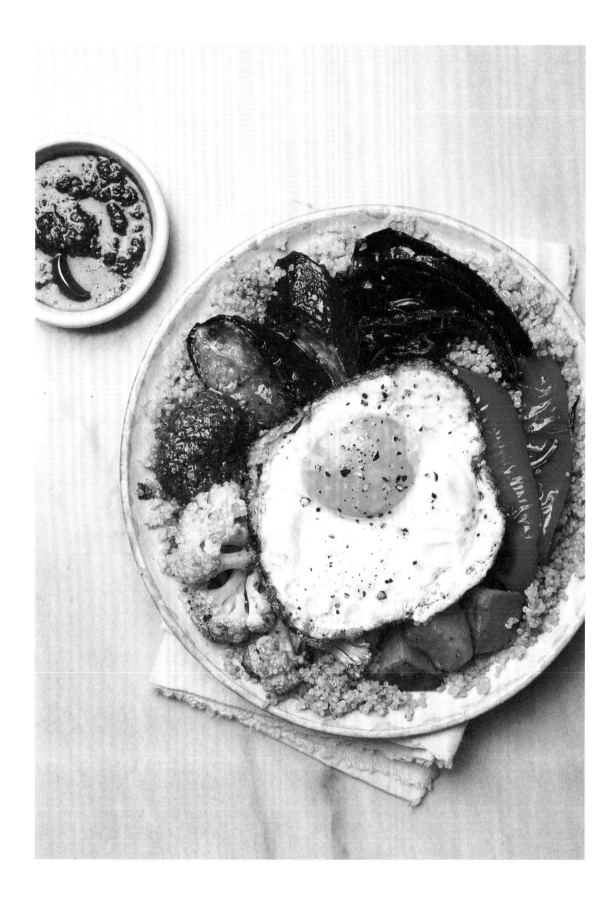

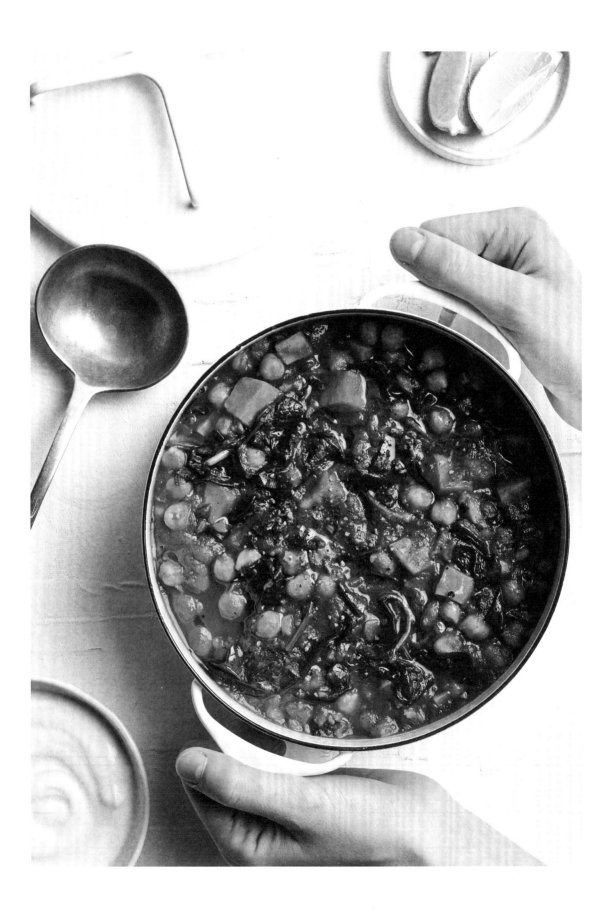

One-Pot Sweet Potato, Spinach, and Chickpea Stew

This is a tasty vegetarian meal you can have on Meatless Mondays or whenever you find yourself craving a simple, nutritious dinner. Initially, I made it as a filling for another recipe, but I couldn't resist eating it all on its own! This stew is buttery and vibrant, and the garnishes of yogurt and lime wedges add a touch of acidity and tanginess to balance the flavours.

¼ cup (60 mL) ghee, Plain Jane Ghee (page 271), or virgin coconut oil, divided

1 small yellow onion, diced

1 clove garlic, minced

1 (½-inch/1 cm) piece of fresh ginger, peeled and minced

1 teaspoon (5 mL) ground coriander

1 teaspoon (5 mL) ground cumin

1 teaspoon (5 mL) garam masala

1 teaspoon (5 mL) sea salt

Pinch of chili powder

1 can (28 ounces/796 mL) crushed tomatoes

1 medium sweet potato, peeled and diced into ½-inch (1 cm) cubes (about 2 to 2½ cups/500 to 625 mL)

2 cups (500 mL) canned chickpeas, drained and rinsed

¾ cup (175 mL) water

4 cups (1 L) packed baby spinach

To Serve

Plain full-fat yogurt or plain coconut yogurt

Lime wedges

1. In a large Dutch oven or a heavy-bottomed pot with a tight-fitting lid over medium heat, melt 2 tablespoons (30 mL) of the ghee. Add the onion, garlic, and ginger. Cook, stirring occasionally, until softened, 7 to 8 minutes.

2. Add the coriander, cumin, garam masala, salt, and chili powder. Stir to combine. Cook for 1 minute until fragrant.

3. Add the tomatoes, sweet potato, chickpeas, and water. Stir to combine. Bring to a boil, then reduce the heat to medium. Cover and cook until the sweet potatoes are fork-tender, 30 to 35 minutes. Remove the lid and add the spinach. Cook for 5 more minutes, uncovered, until the filling thickens and the spinach wilts.

4. Remove from the heat. Gently stir in the remaining 2 tablespoons (30 mL) ghee. Serve with yogurt and lime wedges.

◆ **Dairy-Free:** Serve with plain coconut yogurt instead of plain full-fat yogurt.
Vegan: Use virgin coconut oil instead of ghee. Use coconut yogurt instead of dairy yogurt.

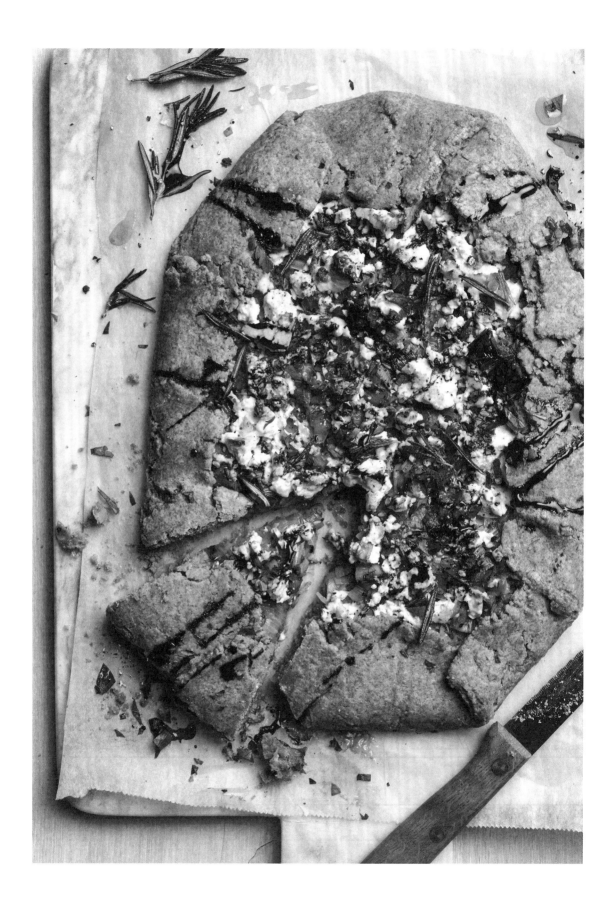

Bone Broth Braised Leek and Goat Cheese Galette

I made this nutrient-dense galette with a sweet and savoury leek filling and gave it a tangy goat cheese twist! The leeks are slow braised in bone broth and become so soft that they melt in the mouth. You can make the dough up to three days ahead and store it in the fridge. When you are rolling out the dough, don't worry if it does not form a perfect oval—galettes are meant to look a bit rustic.

Crust

2 cups (500 mL) sprouted or light spelt flour or 1:1 gluten-free all-purpose flour (not packed)

1 teaspoon (5 mL) sea salt

½ cup (125 mL) cold ghee or Plain Jane Ghee (page 271)

⅓ cup (75 mL) ice water, more as needed

Leek and Goat Cheese Filling

2 tablespoons (30 mL) ghee or Plain Jane Ghee (page 271)

4 large leeks (white and light green parts only), halved lengthwise and thinly sliced into half-circles (about 6 cups/1.5 L)

¾ cup (175 mL) seasoned organic chicken broth or Chicken Bone Broth (page 272)

1 tablespoon (15 mL) chopped fresh rosemary leaves

Sea salt and black pepper, to taste

5 ounces (140 g) goat's milk feta cheese, crumbled

1 pasture-raised or organic egg, whisked

To Serve

Extra-virgin olive oil

Balsamic reduction (see Tip)

¼ cup (60 mL) loosely packed chopped fresh flat-leaf parsley

1. Preheat the oven to 400°F (200°C).
2. **Make the Crust** In a food processor, combine the flour and salt. Add the ghee, 1 tablespoon (15 mL) at a time, pulsing to combine before adding more. After adding all of the ghee, the dough should resemble a coarse meal and be slightly darker in colour.
3. Slowly pour in ⅓ cup (75 mL) ice water while pulsing the dough. Add 1 to 2 tablespoons (15 to 30 mL) more ice water, until the dough comes together in a ball. If the dough is still crumbly, add a bit more ice water, until it holds together well.
4. Scrape the dough onto a lightly floured work surface and, using your hands, form it into a thick disc. Wrap the dough tightly with plastic wrap and place it in the fridge while you prepare the filling.
5. **Braise the Leeks** In a large cast-iron skillet over medium heat, melt the ghee. Add the leeks, chicken broth, and rosemary. Cook, stirring occasionally, until the leeks are soft and the liquid has been absorbed, 18 to 20 minutes. Season with salt and pepper.
6. **Assemble the Galette** Place the dough on a large sheet of parchment paper. Place another large sheet of parchment paper on top of the dough. Roll out the dough into a rough 12- × 14-inch (30 × 35 cm) oval shape, about ⅛-inch (3 mm) thick. Remove the top piece of parchment paper. Carefully transfer the parchment paper with the dough onto a baking sheet.

recipe continues

recipe continued

7. Spread the leek mixture over the dough in an even layer, leaving 1 inch (2.5 cm) of space around the border. Sprinkle the crumbled feta over the leek mixture and fold the edges of the dough over the filling, to form a crust. Brush the crust evenly with the whisked egg. Bake until the crust is golden brown, 25 to 30 minutes.
8. To serve, drizzle the galette with olive oil and balsamic reduction. Top with the parsley. Slice and serve warm.

♦ **Tip:** You can buy balsamic reduction at well-stocked grocery stores or make it at home simply by simmering balsamic vinegar until it reduces to a thick, syrupy consistency.
   Gluten-Free: Use gluten-free all-purpose flour instead of sprouted or light spelt flour.

Beetroot Kitchari with Cilantro-Coconut Chutney

Kitchari is a one-pot Indian stew that is warming, grounding, and extremely easy to digest. This dish is excellent for when you feel sluggish and want to give your digestion a break. I've added beets to this kitchari recipe, for an earthy flavour and beautiful colour. It is essential to soak the split mung beans and rice overnight, as this reduces the cooking time and increases digestibility. You can find many of the ingredients at any Indian supermarket.

Beetroot Kitchari

1 cup (250 mL) split yellow mung beans, soaked in room-temperature water for at least 8 hours, drained, and rinsed

1 cup (250 mL) basmati rice, soaked in room-temperature water for at least 8 hours, drained, and rinsed

4 cups (1 L) seasoned organic vegetable broth

6 cups (1.5 L) water, divided, more as needed

1 bay leaf

3 tablespoons (45 mL) ghee, Plain Jane Ghee (page 271), or virgin coconut oil

1 teaspoon (5 mL) black mustard seeds

1 small yellow onion, diced

1 clove garlic, minced

1 (1-inch/2.5 cm) piece of fresh ginger, peeled and minced

1 teaspoon (5 mL) ground turmeric

½ teaspoon (2 mL) ground coriander

½ teaspoon (2 mL) ground cumin

½ teaspoon (2 mL) black pepper

¾ teaspoon (4 mL) cinnamon

¼ teaspoon (1 mL) ground cardamom

¼ teaspoon (1 mL) ground cloves

4 small red beets, scrubbed, peeled, and grated

2 teaspoons (10 mL) sea salt

Cilantro-Coconut Chutney

¼ cup (60 mL) raw cashews, soaked in room-temperature water for at least 8 hours, drained, and rinsed

2 cups (500 mL) packed fresh cilantro leaves and stems

½ cup (125 mL) frozen young coconut meat, thawed

3 tablespoons (45 mL) fresh lemon juice

1 teaspoon (5 mL) coconut sugar

1 teaspoon (5 mL) sea salt

¼ cup (60 mL) water

1. **Make the Beetroot Kitchari** In a large Dutch oven or a heavy-bottomed pot with a tight-fitting lid, add the soaked mung beans and rice, vegetable broth, 4 cups (1 L) of the water, and bay leaf. Bring to a boil, then reduce the heat to medium. Simmer, covered, until most of the liquid is absorbed and the rice is tender, about 1 hour. If the pot starts to get dry, add more water as needed.
2. Meanwhile, in a medium skillet over medium-high heat, melt the ghee. Add the mustard seeds and cook, stirring often, until they start to pop, 1 to 2 minutes. Add the onion and cook, stirring occasionally, until softened, about 5 minutes. Add the garlic and ginger and cook for 1 minute.
3. Reduce the heat to medium-low. Add the turmeric, coriander, cumin, pepper, cinnamon, cardamom, and cloves. Toast the spices for 3 minutes, stirring frequently, until fragrant.
4. Add the spice mixture to the bean and rice mixture, using a spatula to scrape out the pan.

recipe continues

5. Add the grated beets, salt, and the remaining 2 cups (500 mL) water to the mixture. Stir to combine. Bring to a boil, then reduce the heat to medium. Cook for 20 minutes, covered, stirring occasionally, until the rice is starting to fall apart and the texture is like a thick stew, about 20 minutes. If you prefer a soupier consistency, you can add a bit more broth or water to thin it. Discard the bay leaf.

6. **Make the Cilantro-Coconut Chutney** In a food processor or a high-speed blender, combine the cashews, cilantro, coconut meat, lemon juice, coconut sugar, salt, and water. Blend on high speed until smooth, 15 to 20 seconds.

7. To serve, ladle the Beetroot Kitchari into bowls. Serve with Cilantro-Coconut Chutney.

◆ **Vegan:** Use virgin coconut oil instead of ghee.

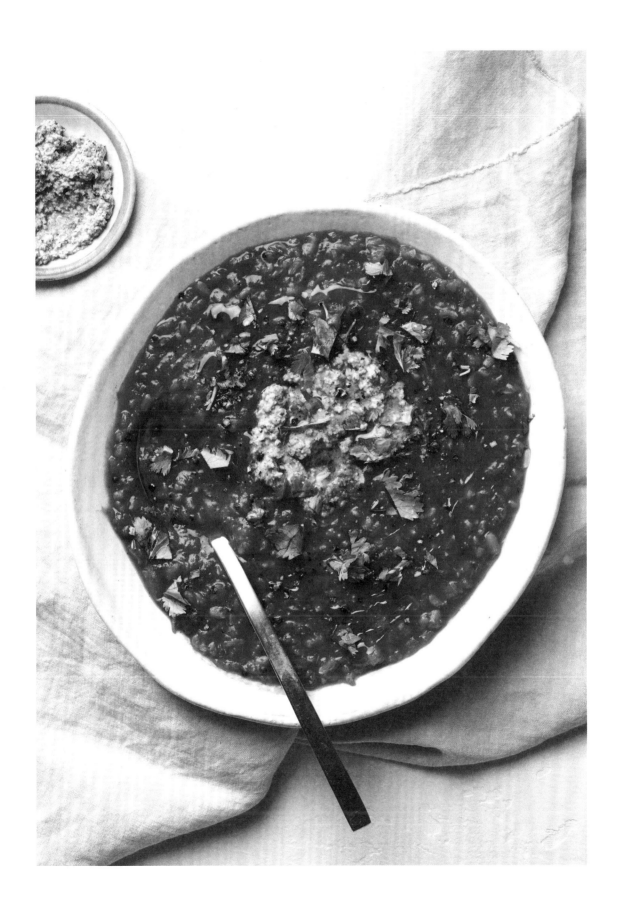

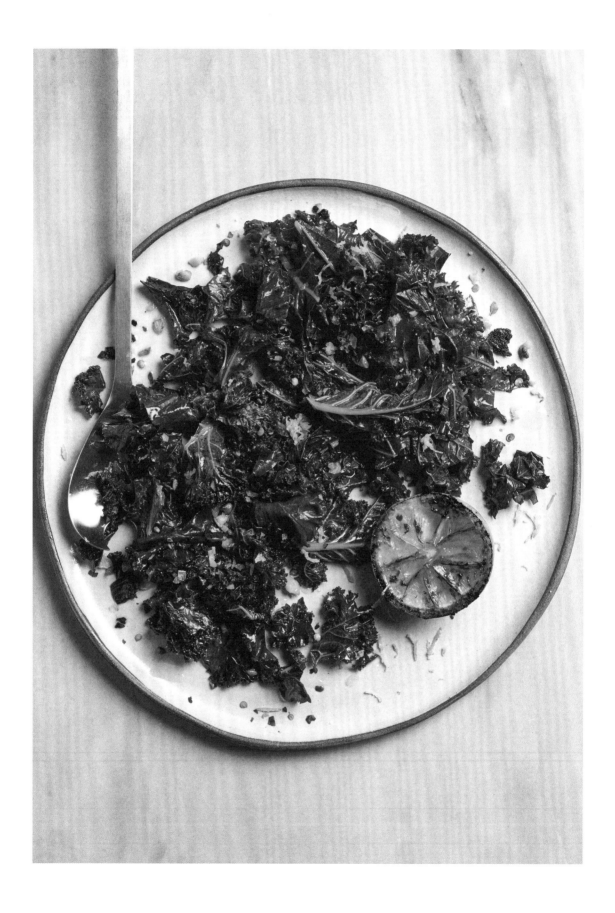

Dairy-Free ◆ Gluten-Free ◆ Grain-Free ◆ Nut-Free ◆ Keto-Friendly
◆ Paleo-Friendly ◆ Vegan Option ◆ Vegetarian ◆ *Serves 2 to 4 as a side*

Spicy Garlicky Wilted Greens

I make this delicious side dish whenever I want to add some extra greens to a meal. I learned this simple Italian cooking technique from a friend in New York. Traditionally, olive oil is used to sauté the greens, but I prefer to use ghee or avocado oil for its high smoke point and instead add the olive oil at the end as a finishing oil for flavour.

2 tablespoons (30 mL) ghee, Plain Jane Ghee (page 271), or duck fat

4 cloves garlic, thinly sliced

6 cups (1.5 L) packed chopped curly kale, stems and ribs removed

½ teaspoon (2 mL) red chili flakes

1 tablespoon (15 mL) fresh lemon juice

1 teaspoon (5 mL) lemon zest, to serve

Flaky sea salt, to taste

Extra-virgin olive oil, to serve

1. In a large skillet over medium-high heat, heat the ghee. Add the sliced garlic and cook until it just starts to brown, about 1 minute.

2. Add the kale and chili flakes. Using tongs, toss to coat. Sauté, tossing often, until the greens are wilted and tender, 4 to 5 minutes.

3. Add the lemon juice and toss to combine. Remove from the heat.

4. Transfer to a small serving platter. Sprinkle with the lemon zest and flaky sea salt. Finish with a drizzle of olive oil.

◆ **Vegan:** Use avocado oil instead of ghee.

Farinata with Olives, Rosemary, and Sun-Dried Tomatoes

Farinata is a chickpea flatbread that originated in Italy. I first tried the lesser-known variation, *fainá*, while backpacking in Argentina in my early twenties. It would be served with deep-dish pizza, but I loved it on its own and would eat it plain with some good olive oil on top. I started making it at home and experimented with different toppings—this Mediterranean-inspired version is my favourite. It makes for a light and healthy vegetarian lunch served with Chopped Avocado Caprese Salad (page 102).

2 cups (500 mL) chickpea flour

3 cups (750 mL) warm water

½ cup (125 mL) grated pecorino cheese

2 teaspoons (10 mL) sea salt

1 teaspoon (5 mL) black pepper

¼ cup (60 mL) ghee or Plain Jane Ghee (page 271), melted, more for the pan

1 tablespoon + 1½ teaspoons (22 mL) chopped fresh rosemary leaves

⅓ cup (75 mL) pitted Kalamata olives, cut in half

⅓ cup (75 mL) sun-dried tomatoes, thinly sliced

½ small red onion, thinly sliced

To Serve

¼ cup (60 mL) loosely packed chopped fresh flat-leaf parsley

Extra-virgin olive oil

Freshly ground black pepper

1. Preheat the oven to 450°F (230°C). Grease the sides and base of a large cast-iron skillet with a bit of ghee.

2. In a large bowl, add the chickpea flour. Slowly whisk in the warm water, until the mixture is completely smooth. Add the pecorino, salt, and pepper. Cover with a clean kitchen towel and let sit at room temperature for 30 minutes.

3. Add the melted ghee to the batter. Whisk to combine.

4. Place the empty cast-iron skillet in the oven to preheat for 5 minutes. Carefully pour the batter evenly into the hot skillet. Scatter the rosemary, olives, sun-dried tomatoes, and red onion over the batter.

5. Return the skillet to the oven and bake until the batter is set and lightly golden around the edges, 16 to 20 minutes.

6. Set the oven to broil. Broil until the top is golden brown, 1 to 2 minutes.

7. To serve, cut into slices and sprinkle with the parsley. Drizzle with olive oil and finish with pepper. Serve warm.

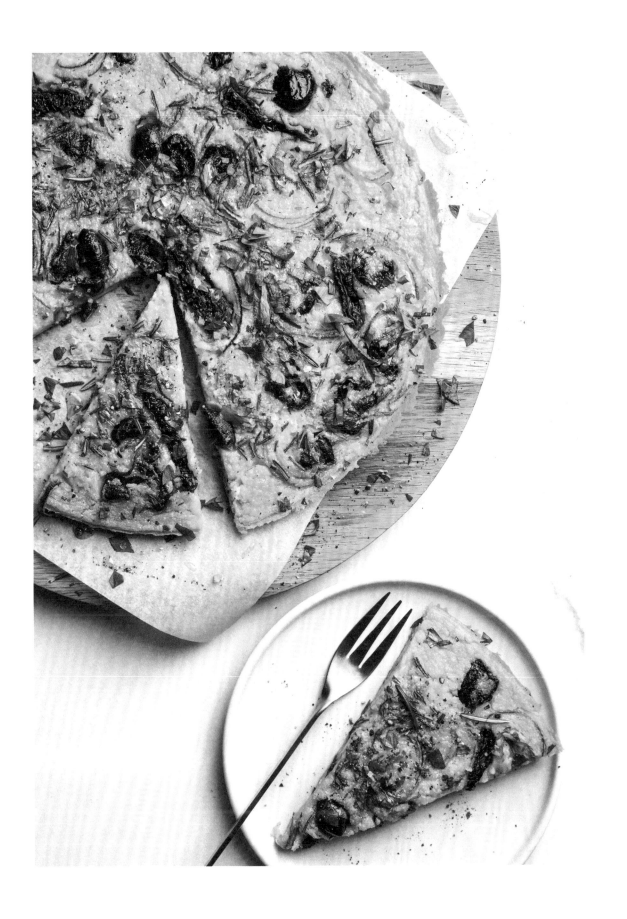

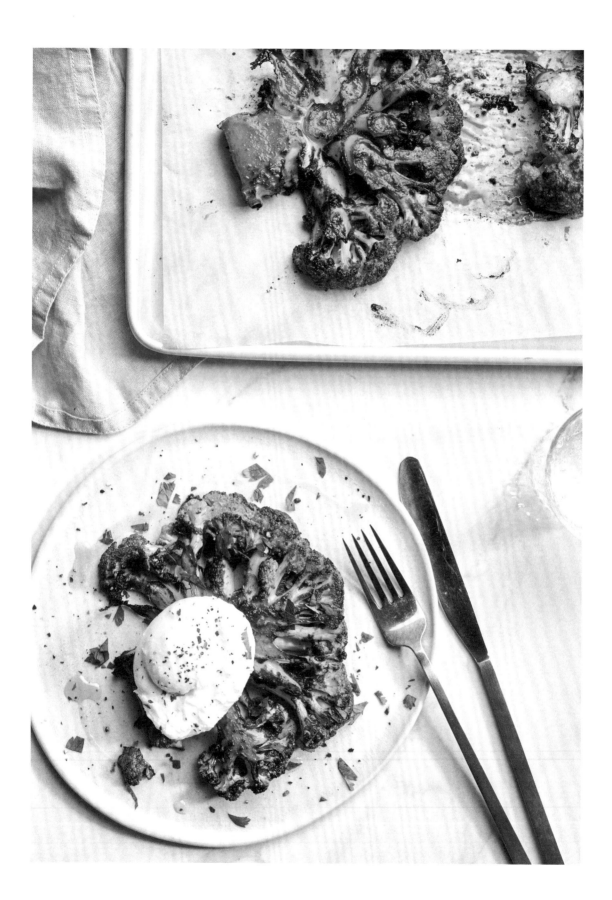

Dairy-Free ◆ Gluten-Free ◆ Grain-Free ◆ Nut-Free
◆ Paleo-Friendly ◆ Vegan Option ◆ Vegetarian ◆ *Serves 2*

◆ Harissa Roasted Cauliflower Steaks

I make this recipe whenever I am in the mood for a satisfying plant-based meal—it is surprisingly filling and utterly delicious! The sharp, sweet, and spicy cauliflower is full of flavour and caramelized to perfection. Harissa paste is available at specialty food shops, or you can substitute any chili-based hot sauce. You can use the leftover cauliflower to make cauliflower rice to serve with Slow-Cooked Butter Chicken (page 121). Cook the Poached Eggs (page 268) just before serving.

1 head of cauliflower

2 tablespoons (30 mL) ghee or Plain Jane Ghee (page 271), at room temperature

1 tablespoon + 1½ teaspoons (22 mL) mild harissa paste or chili-based hot sauce

1½ teaspoons (7 mL) pomegranate molasses

Sea salt and black pepper, to taste

To Serve

2 Poached Eggs (page 268)

Red chili flakes (optional)

Chopped fresh flat-leaf parsley

Extra-virgin olive oil

Lime wedges

1. Preheat the oven to 400°F (200°C).

2. With the cauliflower resting upright on a cutting board, slice it in half down the middle. Cut a 1-inch (2.5 cm) thick slice from each side of the middle cut. Lay the 2 slices of cauliflower flat on the cutting board. Using a knife, carefully remove the outer leaves and stem.

3. In a small bowl, whisk together the ghee, harissa, and pomegranate molasses.

4. In a large bowl, add the slices of cauliflower and harissa mixture. Using your hands, massage the harissa mixture all over the cauliflower. Season with salt and pepper. Carefully transfer the cauliflower slices to an unlined baking sheet. Roast until the edges are golden brown and the core is tender when pricked with the tip of a knife, 35 to 40 minutes, turning the cauliflower at the 25-minute mark.

5. To serve, divide the cauliflower steaks between 2 plates. Top each with a Poached Egg. Garnish with chili flakes (if using), parsley, and a drizzle of olive oil. Serve with lime wedges.

◆ **Vegan:** Use virgin coconut oil instead of ghee. Skip the poached eggs.

◆ Roasted Vegetables with Tahini Drizzle

The secret to achieving golden brown roasted vegetables is spreading them out evenly on a baking sheet with space between each piece. This prevents them from steaming, rather than browning, and makes them delightfully crispy around the edges. This simple side dish has many different colours and textures, which makes for a beautiful presentation. The tahini drizzle on top is the best part! I prefer thinner tahini because it is easy to drizzle. If your tahini is on the thicker side, simply add more melted ghee to thin it to a pourable consistency.

½ head of purple cabbage, core removed and sliced into ½-inch (1 cm) thick wedges

1 pound (450 g) multicoloured carrots, scrubbed and sliced in half lengthwise

3 yellow beets, peeled and roughly chopped

1 pound (450 g) Brussels sprouts, ends trimmed and cut in half

8 ounces (225 g) Jerusalem artichokes, scrubbed and roughly chopped

10 cloves garlic

¼ cup (60 mL) avocado oil

Sea salt and black pepper, to taste

5 sprigs of fresh thyme

⅓ cup (75 mL) tahini

3 tablespoons (45 mL) ghee or Plain Jane Ghee (page 271), melted

2 tablespoons (30 mL) sesame seeds

1. Position racks in the upper and lower thirds of the oven. Preheat the oven to 425°F (220°C).
2. In a large bowl, add the cabbage, carrots, beets, Brussels sprouts, artichokes, and garlic. Toss with the avocado oil, salt, and pepper.
3. Arrange the vegetables on 2 unlined baking sheets. Spread them out in a single layer, ensuring that there is 1 inch (2.5 cm) of space between each piece. Top with the thyme sprigs. Bake for 40 to 45 minutes, rotating the baking sheets front to back and top rack to bottom rack halfway through cooking. Discard the thyme sprigs.
4. In a small bowl, whisk together the tahini, melted ghee, salt, and pepper.
5. To serve, transfer the vegetables to a serving platter. Drizzle with the tahini mixture and sprinkle with the sesame seeds.

◆ **Vegan:** Use coconut oil instead of ghee.

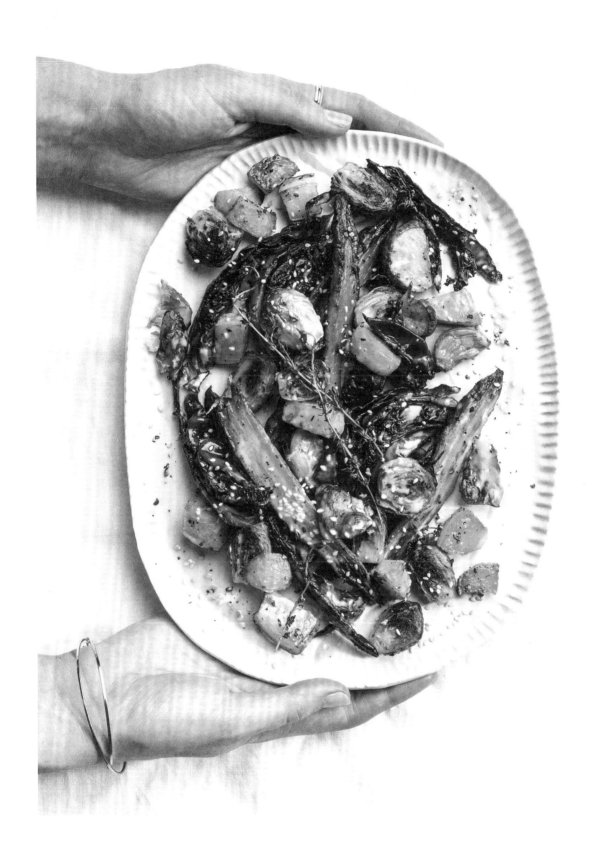

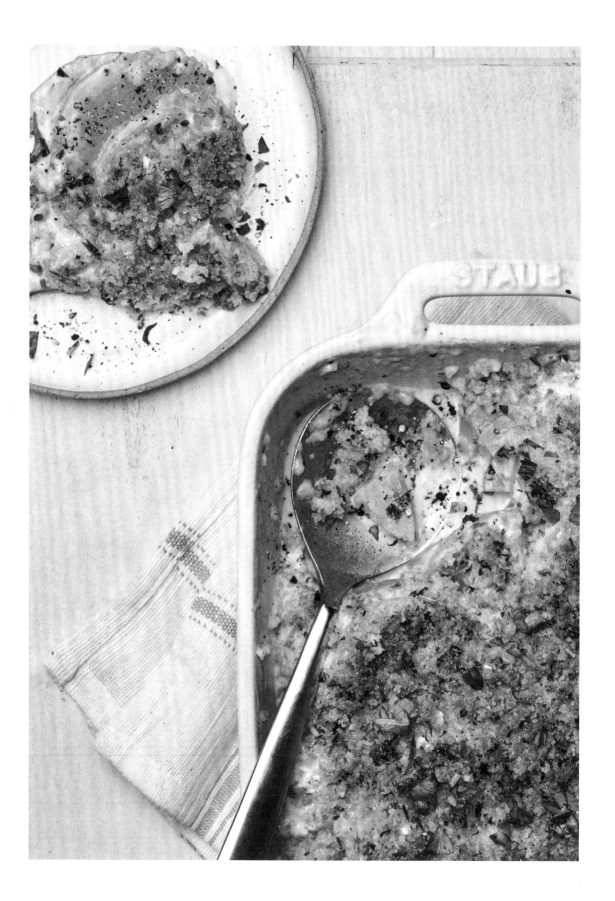

◆ Squash Gratin with Buttered Bread Crumbs

This recipe is a crowd-pleasing side dish for Thanksgiving or any special occasion—it tastes like an indulgent treat! I really enjoy the buttery flavour, the soft texture of the cooked squash, and the crunch of the bread crumbs. This is delicious served with Pistachio-Crusted Rack of Lamb with Pomegranate Butter Glaze (page 139) and green beans.

Squash Gratin

1 tablespoon (15 mL) ghee, Plain Jane Ghee (page 271), or virgin coconut oil, more for the baking dish

2½ cups (625 mL) canned full-fat coconut milk

1 cup (250 mL) seasoned organic chicken broth or Chicken Bone Broth (page 272)

1 tablespoon (15 mL) Dijon mustard

Sea salt and black pepper, to taste

1 butternut squash (about 3 pounds/1.35 kg), peeled, halved, and seeded

1½ cups (375 mL) grated pecorino cheese, divided

Buttered Bread Crumbs

2 tablespoons (30 mL) ghee, Plain Jane Ghee (page 271), or virgin coconut oil

¾ cup (175 mL) panko or gluten-free bread crumbs

¼ cup (60 mL) loosely packed chopped fresh flat-leaf parsley, more to garnish

Sea salt and pepper, to taste

1. Preheat the oven to 400°F (200°C). Grease the base and sides of an 11- × 7-inch (2 L) baking dish with a bit of ghee.

2. **Make the Squash Gratin** In a medium saucepan over medium-low heat, whisk together the ghee, coconut milk, chicken broth, mustard, salt, and pepper. Bring to a boil over high heat. Reduce the heat to medium and simmer, stirring frequently, until slightly thickened, 10 to 12 minutes.

3. Cut the butternut squash into ⅓-inch (8 mm) thick half-moon slices. Place a layer of squash on the bottom of the baking dish, arranging the slices so that they fit together as tightly as possible. Season with salt and pepper. Sprinkle with ½ cup (125 mL) of the pecorino.

4. Add a second layer of squash to the baking dish. Season with salt and pepper and sprinkle with ½ cup (125 mL) pecorino. Add a third layer of squash to the baking dish. Season with salt and pepper. Pour the coconut milk mixture over the squash. Cover the dish tightly with foil and bake until the squash is fork-tender, 50 to 60 minutes.

5. **Make the Buttered Bread Crumbs** In a medium skillet over medium heat, melt the ghee. Add the bread crumbs and stir to coat. Cook, stirring occasionally, until the crumbs darken slightly, 4 to 5 minutes. Add the parsley, salt and pepper. Stir to combine.

6. Remove the foil from the dish and sprinkle the remaining ½ cup (125 mL) pecorino on top. Spoon the Buttered Bread Crumbs over the gratin. Bake, uncovered, for 5 to 10 more minutes. Cool for 10 minutes before serving. Garnish with fresh parsley.

◆ **Gluten-Free:** Use gluten-free bread crumbs instead of panko.

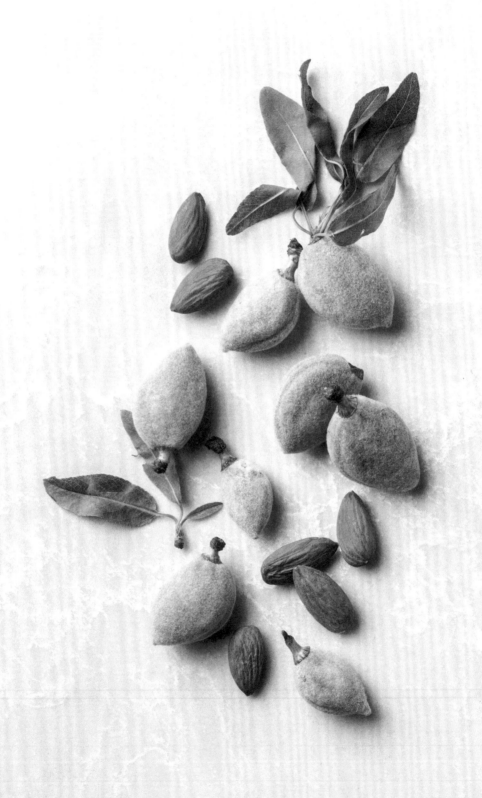

Snacks and Small Bites

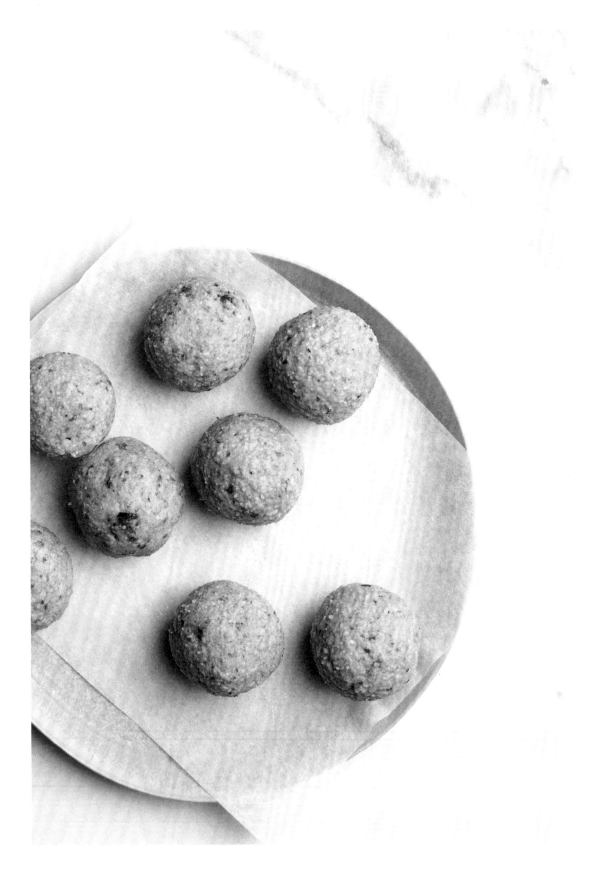

◆ Tahini-Coconut Fat Balls

These delicious fat balls are the perfect snack to have on hand for mid-morning or afternoon hunger cravings. As the name suggests, they are full of energizing fats from coconut, cashews, almonds, sunflower seeds, tahini, and hemp seeds. They have an incredible, nutty flavour and are lightly sweetened with dates. I like to always have a batch in my fridge or freezer for snacking on.

1 cup (250 mL) unsweetened shredded coconut

½ cup (125 mL) raw cashews

½ cup (125 mL) raw whole almonds

½ cup (125 mL) raw sunflower seeds

¼ cup (60 mL) tahini

3 tablespoons (45 mL) hulled hemp seeds

3 soft Medjool dates, pitted

3 tablespoons (45 mL) virgin coconut oil

¼ teaspoon (1 mL) cinnamon

Pinch of ground cardamom

Pinch of sea salt

1. In a food processor, combine the coconut, cashews, almonds, and sunflower seeds. Blend on high speed until ground into a coarse meal, 15 to 20 seconds.

2. Add the tahini, hemp seeds, dates, coconut oil, cinnamon, cardamom, and salt. Blend again on high speed until the mixture sticks together when squished in the palm of your hand, about 10 seconds. The mixture should feel oily.

3. Scoop 1 heaping tablespoon (18 mL) of the mixture and, using your hands, roll it into a ball. Repeat with the rest of the mixture. Place the fat balls, in a single layer, in an airtight container and freeze for at least 1 hour to harden. Store in the fridge for up to 1 month or in the freezer for up to 3 months.

Raw Chipotle Spiced Coconut Chips

My friend Tara Tomulka, a holistic nutritionist and founder of Rawcology, developed this recipe. These spicy, smoky coconut chips taste just like coconut bacon—they are the perfect fat-fuelled savoury snack to bring with you to work. Coconut chips contain medium-chain triglycerides (MCTs), which provide a quick source of energy for the body and mind. Since the chips are raw, you can use either a food dehydrator or a conventional oven on its lowest temperature setting for this recipe. This recipe also can easily be halved to make a smaller portion.

3 tablespoons (45 mL) gluten-free tamari or coconut aminos

1 teaspoon (5 mL) apple cider vinegar

1 teaspoon (5 mL) chipotle powder

1 teaspoon (5 mL) ground cumin

1 teaspoon (5 mL) smoked paprika

½ teaspoon (2 mL) sea salt

4 cups (1 L) unsweetened coconut flakes

1. If you are using an oven, position racks in the upper and lower thirds of the oven. Preheat the oven to 150°F (65°C) and line 2 baking sheets with parchment paper. If you are using a food dehydrator, turn on the machine and set the temperature to 115°F (46°C).

2. In a small bowl, whisk together the tamari, apple cider vinegar, chipotle powder, cumin, smoked paprika, and salt.

3. In a large bowl, add the coconut flakes. Add the spice mixture to the coconut flakes and toss until all of the flakes are thoroughly coated.

4. If you are using an oven, spread the coconut chips evenly on the prepared baking sheets. Dehydrate in the oven until the coconut chips are crispy like potato chips, 2½ to 3 hours. If you are using a food dehydrator, spread the coconut chips evenly on the dehydrator trays. Dehydrate until the coconut chips are crispy like potato chips, 4 to 5 hours. Store in an airtight container at room temperature for up to 3 weeks.

◆ **Paleo-Friendly and Keto-Friendly:** Use coconut aminos instead of gluten-free tamari.

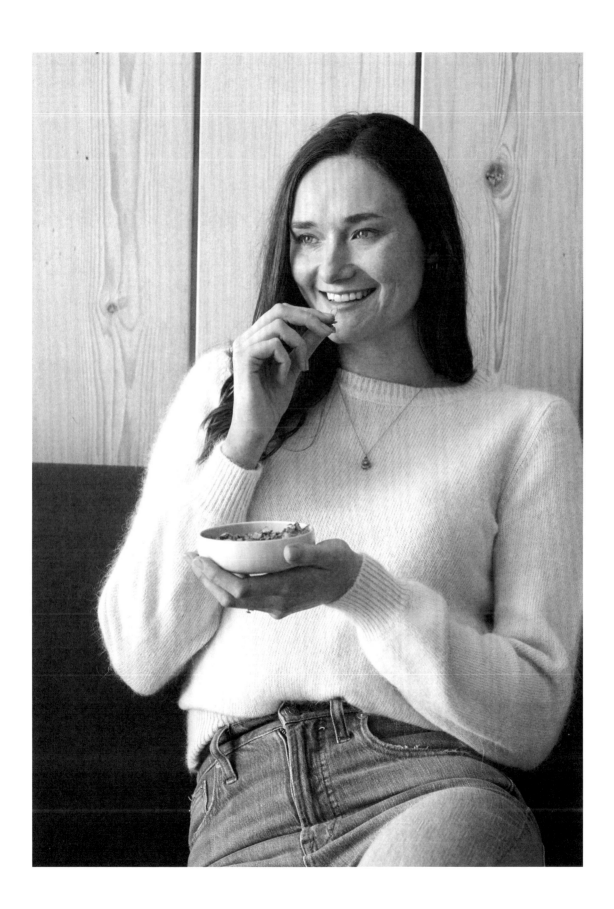

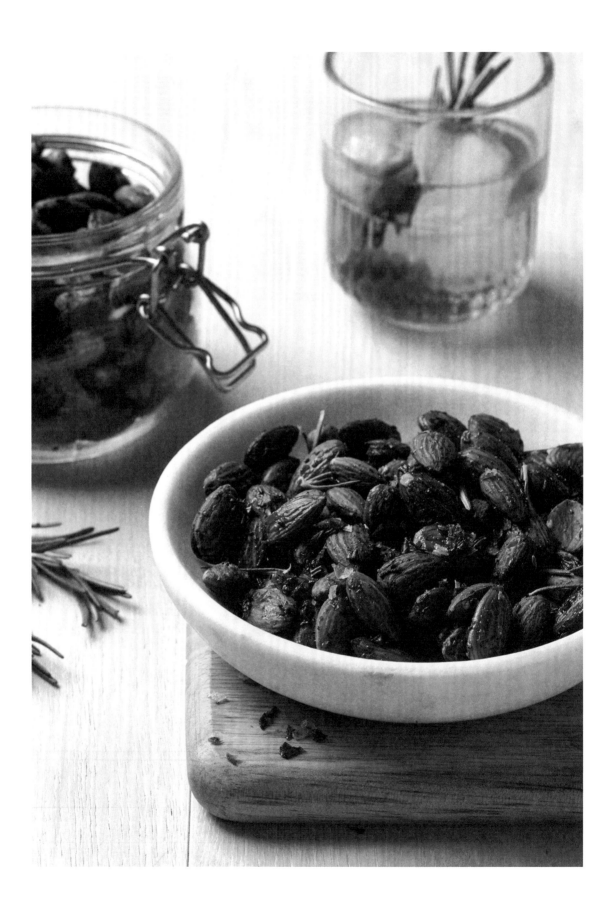

◆ Rosemary Roasted Almonds

These almonds were adapted from a recipe by our former community manager, Julia Gibson. Almonds are a great source of heart- and brain-loving monounsaturated fats that help lower cholesterol in the body. These almonds have an herbaceous, woody flavour with a hint of sweetness and spice. I like making them as a snack to bring to work, but they are equally great served as an appetizer.

1 tablespoon + 1½ teaspoons (22 mL) melted ghee or Plain Jane Ghee (page 271)

2 tablespoons (30 mL) pure maple syrup

3 cups (750 mL) raw whole almonds

6 sprigs of fresh rosemary, leaves only, roughly chopped

½ teaspoon (2 mL) cayenne pepper

½ teaspoon (2 mL) sea salt

1. Preheat the oven to 350°F (180°C). Line a baking sheet with parchment paper.
2. In a large bowl, mix together the ghee and maple syrup. Add the almonds, rosemary, cayenne, and salt. Toss to combine.
3. Spread the almonds evenly in a single layer on the prepared baking sheet. Bake until the almonds are crunchy and have some darker colour on them, 12 to 15 minutes, stirring once halfway through baking time. Store in an airtight container in the fridge for up to 2 weeks.

◆ **Vegan:** Use virgin coconut oil instead of ghee.

◆ Seedy Almond Pulp Crackers

After making a batch of Nut Milk (page 273), I make these crackers with the leftover nutrient-rich almond pulp to not let it go to waste. Since these crackers are baked at a lower oven temperature, you can use olive oil in them without the risk of it oxidizing in the oven. The seeds add healthy omega-3 fatty acids, making these crackers a powerhouse of anti-inflammatory goodness. They are the perfect grain-free dipping vessel for Kalamata Olive Tapenade (page 200) or Whipped Feta Spread (page 208).

1 cup (250 mL) packed almond pulp (see page 263)

1 tablespoon (15 mL) golden flax seeds

1 tablespoon (15 mL) white sesame seeds

1 tablespoon (15 mL) white chia seeds

1 sprig of fresh rosemary, leaves only, roughly chopped

½ teaspoon (2 mL) baking soda

2 tablespoons (30 mL) extra-virgin olive oil

¼ teaspoon (1 mL) sea salt

1. Preheat the oven to 300°F (150°C). Line a baking sheet with parchment paper.

2. In a large bowl, combine the almond pulp, flax seeds, sesame seeds, chia seeds, rosemary, baking soda, olive oil, and salt. Using your hands, form the dough into one solid mass and transfer it to the prepared baking sheet.

3. Place a second sheet of parchment paper over the dough. Using a rolling pin, roll out the dough to a rectangular shape about ⅛-inch (3 mm) thick. Remove the top sheet of parchment paper. Using a pizza cutter, carefully slice the dough into 1½-inch (4 cm) squares. Using a fork, prick each square three times. Bake for 30 minutes. Remove from the oven and carefully separate and flip the crackers, then bake until they are crispy and lightly browned, 15 to 20 minutes. Let cool completely. Store the crackers in an airtight container in the fridge for up to 7 days.

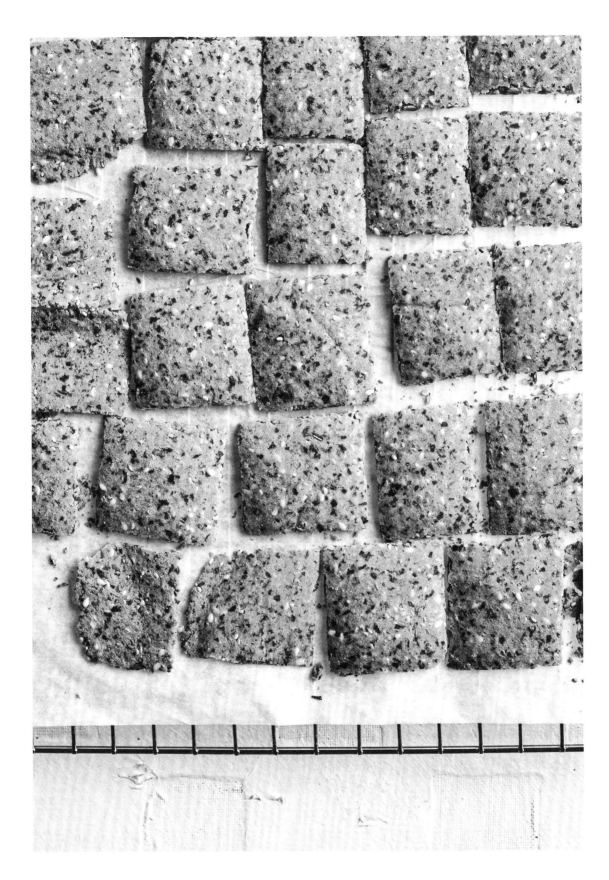

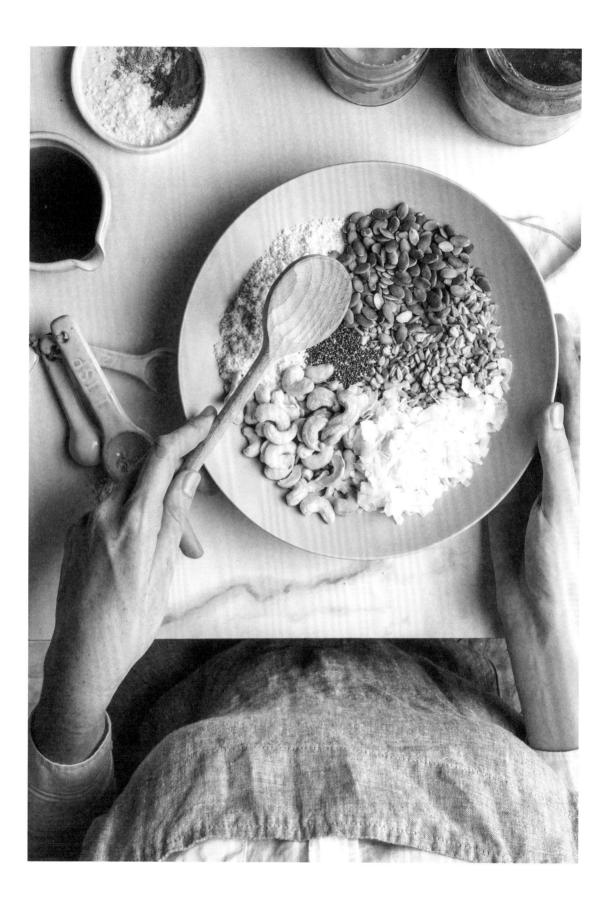

◆ Chewy Grainless Granola Bars

These grain-free granola bars are chewy, sweet, and salty, which makes them totally addictive! They are full of good fats, protein, and fibre from a variety of nuts and seeds, which makes them a very satiating snack that will curb your hunger for hours. To prevent the bars from crumbling, be sure to grind the nuts and seeds into a fine meal (similar in texture to almond flour) and always cool the bars for at least 1 hour after they come out of the oven before slicing.

1½ cups (375 mL) raw sunflower seeds

1 cup (250 mL) raw cashews

1 cup (250 mL) raw pumpkin seeds

1 cup (250 mL) unsweetened coconut flakes

½ cup (125 mL) super-fine blanched almond flour

1 tablespoon (15 mL) black chia seeds

½ teaspoon (2 mL) cinnamon

¼ teaspoon (1 mL) ground cardamom

½ teaspoon (2 mL) coarse sea salt

½ cup (125 mL) melted ghee or Plain Jane Ghee (page 271)

½ cup (125 mL) pure maple syrup

¼ cup (60 mL) natural almond butter or Homemade Almond Butter (page 275)

1 teaspoon (5 mL) pure vanilla extract or ½ teaspoon (2 mL) pure vanilla powder

1. Position a rack in the middle of the oven. Preheat the oven to 300°F (150°C). Line a 12½- × 8½-inch (3.5 L) glass baking dish with parchment paper.

2. In a food processor, combine the sunflower seeds, cashews, pumpkin seeds, and coconut flakes. Pulse until the nuts and seeds are ground into a fine meal. Transfer the mixture to a large bowl. Add the almond flour, chia seeds, cinnamon, cardamom, and salt. Stir to combine.

3. In a medium bowl, mix together the melted ghee, maple syrup, almond butter, and vanilla. Pour the ghee mixture into the ground seed and nut mixture. Stir well to combine. At this point, the mixture should be sticky and hold its shape when squeezed in your hand.

4. Scrape the mixture into the prepared baking dish. Using your fingers, press the mixture evenly into the bottom of the dish. Bake until the edges are golden brown, 35 to 45 minutes. Let cool for at least 1 hour before slicing. Store the bars in an airtight container in the fridge for up to 1 month or in the freezer for up to 3 months.

◆ **Paleo-Friendly:** Use pure vanilla powder instead of pure vanilla extract.
Vegan: Use virgin coconut oil instead of ghee.

◆ Turmeric Ghee Popcorn

This is my favourite popcorn to make for movie nights. I first developed the recipe for sampling my turmeric-infused ghee at a farmers market. It was so popular that I still get asked today when I will make it again. With its vibrant yellow hue and buttery flavour, it looks and tastes like movie theatre popcorn. Only instead of artificial colours and flavours, it is made with good old turmeric and ghee! The nutritional yeast adds a cheesy flavour that makes the popcorn super addictive.

1 tablespoon (15 mL) avocado oil

⅔ cup (150 mL) organic popcorn kernels

¼ cup (60 mL) ghee, Plain Jane Ghee (page 271) or coconut oil

1 teaspoon (5 mL) ground turmeric

2 tablespoons (30 mL) nutritional yeast (optional)

Sea salt, to taste

1. In a large, heavy-bottomed pot over medium-high heat, heat the avocado oil. Add 2 or 3 popcorn kernels to the pot and cover with a lid. When the kernels pop, add the remaining popcorn kernels. Cover and give the pot a good shake to coat the kernels in oil. Leave the pot, undisturbed, over the heat while the popcorn pops. When the popping slows to a few seconds between each pop, give the pot a good shake and remove it from the heat.

2. In a small saucepan over low heat, melt the ghee. Add the turmeric and stir to combine. Pour the turmeric ghee over the popcorn.

3. Add the nutritional yeast (if using) and salt. Shake well to combine. Transfer to a large bowl and enjoy.

◆ **Vegan:** Use coconut oil instead of ghee.

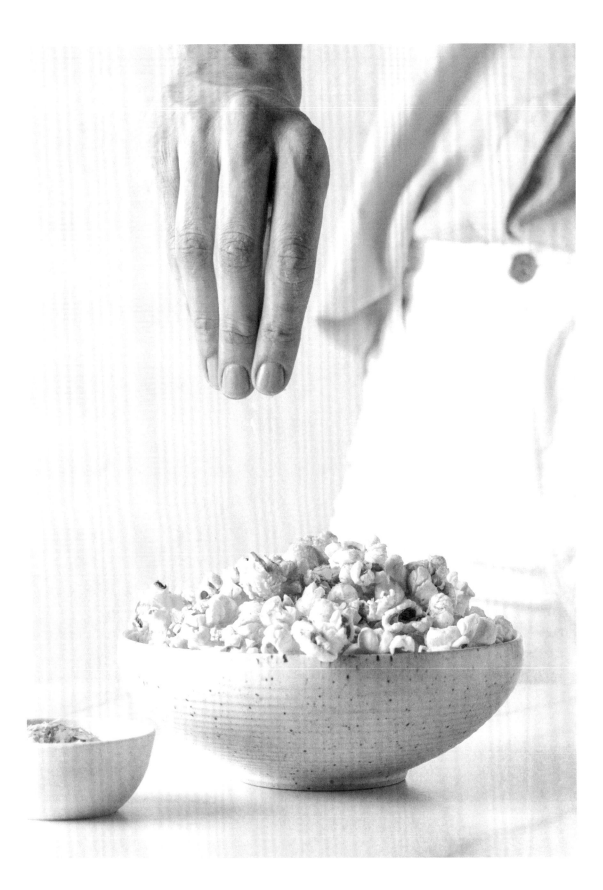

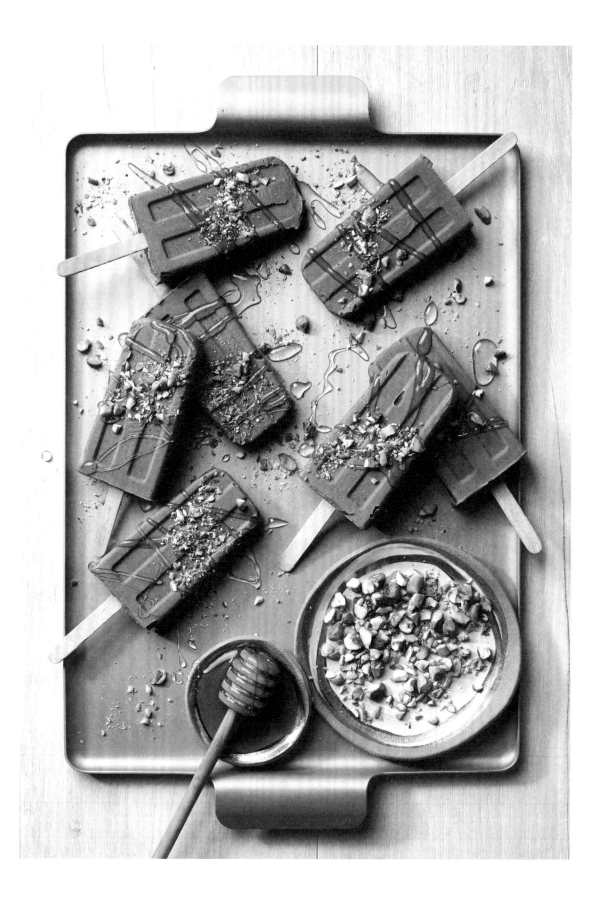

Dreamy Avocado Fudgesicles

These creamy, dreamy fudgesicles are the perfect treat for a summer day. They get their creaminess from coconut milk, almond butter, and avocado, which makes them energizing, satiating, and filling. Get creative and top them with a drizzle of honey and chopped pistachios for a bit of crunch, as shown in the photo. This is the perfect fat-fuelled snack, if you ask me!

1 can (14 ounces/398 mL) full-fat coconut milk

10 soft Medjool dates, pitted

1 small avocado, peeled and pitted

3 tablespoons (45 mL) raw cacao powder

2 tablespoons (30 mL) raw liquid honey or pure maple syrup

2 tablespoons (30 mL) natural almond butter or Homemade Almond Butter (page 275)

¼ teaspoon (1 mL) pure vanilla extract or a pinch of pure vanilla powder

Pinch of sea salt

1. In a high-speed blender or a food processor, combine the coconut milk, dates, avocado, cacao powder, honey, almond butter, vanilla, and salt. Blend on high speed, scraping down the sides as needed, until smooth, 20 to 30 seconds.
2. Spoon the mixture into each well of an 8 ice-pop mould. Carefully insert the ice-pop sticks and freeze until solid, at least 4 hours.
3. When ready to serve, run the ice-pop mould under hot water for 5 to 10 seconds and the fudgesicles will easily slide out of the mould. Enjoy immediately. Store any leftover fudgesicles in an airtight container in the freezer for up to 1 month.

◆ **Paleo-Friendly:** Use pure vanilla powder instead of pure vanilla extract.
Vegan: Use pure maple syrup instead of raw honey.

Dairy-Free ◆ Gluten-Free ◆ Grain-Free ◆ Nut-Free ◆ Keto-Friendly ◆ Paleo-Friendly ◆ Vegan Option ◆ *Makes 1 cup (250 mL)*

◆ Kalamata Olive Tapenade

This savoury olive tapenade is a staple in our kitchen for appetizers and snacking alike. It can be made either smooth or chunky, depending on your preference. Enjoy this umami spread on Seedy Almond Pulp Crackers (page 192) or as a dip for crudités. However you enjoy it, you'll be sure to get a healthy dose of anti-inflammatory fats that will keep you looking and feeling your best.

1 clove garlic, minced

¾ cup (175 mL) pitted Kalamata olives

2¼ teaspoons (11 mL) extra-virgin olive oil

1½ teaspoons (7 mL) fresh lemon juice

½ teaspoon (2 mL) rinsed and drained capers

1 anchovy fillet

Pinch of black pepper

1 batch Seedy Almond Pulp Crackers (page 192), for serving

1. In a food processor, combine the garlic, olives, olive oil, lemon juice, capers, anchovy, and pepper. Blend on high speed until the mixture reaches your desired consistency, 10 to 15 seconds.

2. Transfer to a small bowl and serve with Seedy Almond Pulp Crackers. Store the tapenade in an airtight container in the fridge for up to 3 weeks.

◆ **Vegan:** Skip the anchovy fillet.

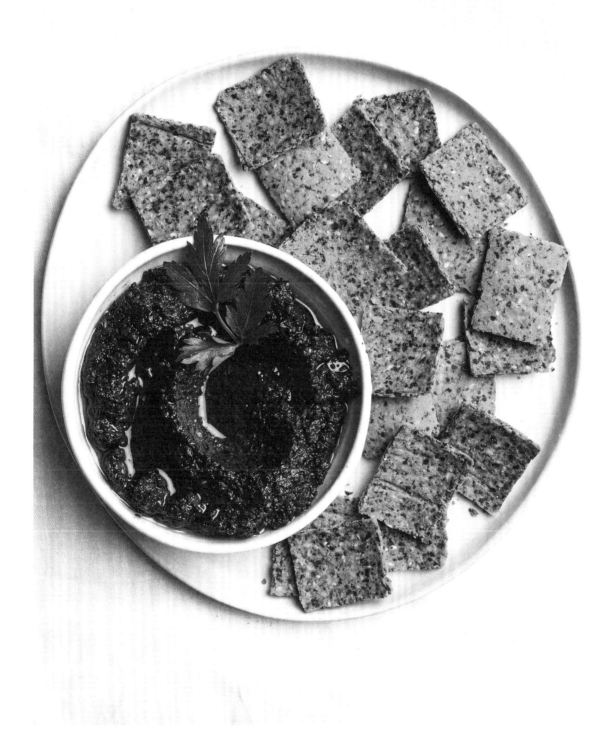

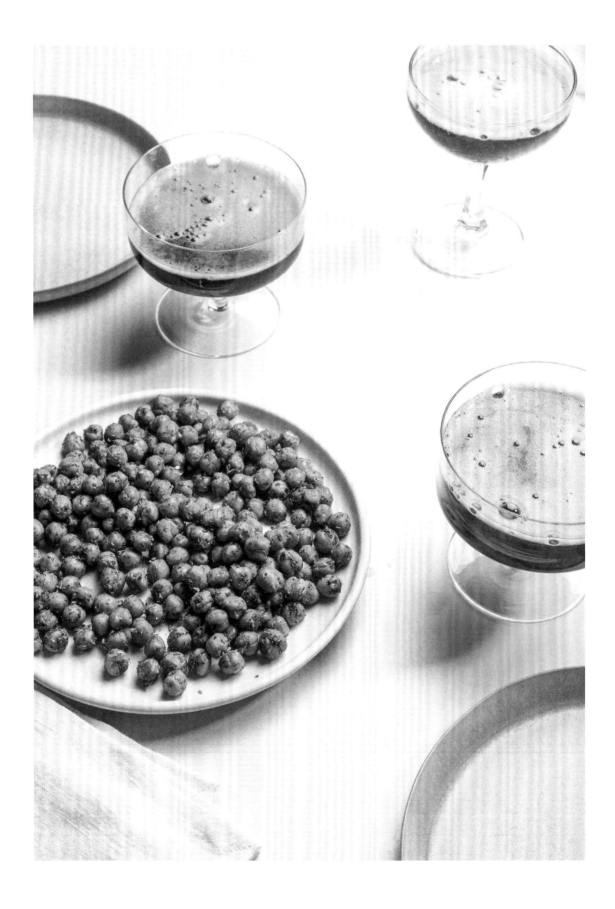

Crispy Za'atar Chickpeas

These roasted chickpeas are crisped to perfection, using avocado oil for its high smoke point and olive oil as a finishing oil for added flavour. The trick to getting them crispy is drying them thoroughly before roasting and leaving space between each chickpea while roasting. These chickpeas are irresistible when served warm out of the oven, topped with flaky sea salt.

2 cups (500 mL) canned chickpeas, drained and rinsed

1 tablespoon (15 mL) avocado oil

½ teaspoon (2 mL) sea salt

1½ teaspoons (7 mL) extra-virgin olive oil

2 tablespoons (30 mL) za'atar

¼ teaspoon (1 mL) flaky sea salt

1. Preheat the oven to 400°F (200°C). Line a baking sheet with parchment paper.
2. Dry the chickpeas thoroughly with a clean kitchen towel or paper towel. Arrange them in a single layer on the towel to air-dry completely for 30 minutes. The drier the chickpeas are, the crispier they will get.
3. In a medium bowl, toss the chickpeas with the avocado oil and salt. Spread the chickpeas evenly in a single layer on the prepared baking sheet, leaving space between each chickpea. Roast until the chickpeas are golden brown and crispy, 25 to 30 minutes, tossing them halfway through baking time.
4. Remove from the oven and add the olive oil, za'atar, and flaky sea salt. Toss to combine. Transfer to a small serving dish and enjoy immediately.

Roasted Plantain Wedges

These roasted plantains are a delicious, easy snack that you can make in under half an hour. Plantain wedges hold their shape well, which makes them great for dipping into Smashed Avocado Butter (page 207) for a healthy snack. I roast them in virgin coconut oil to produce a nostalgic tropical flavour that takes me back to my journey through Kerala in India. You can find plantains at most grocery stores—just be sure to look for ones that have a lot of black markings on the peel, which means they are fully ripened.

3 plantains, peeled and sliced lengthwise into 4 wedges

1 tablespoon (15 mL) melted virgin coconut oil

1 teaspoon (5 mL) garlic powder

¼ teaspoon (1 mL) cayenne pepper

¼ teaspoon (1 mL) sea salt

1 batch Smashed Avocado Butter (page 207), for serving

1. Preheat the oven to 375°F (190°C).
2. In a large bowl, toss the plantain wedges with the melted coconut oil, garlic powder, cayenne, and salt. Spread the wedges in a single layer on an unlined baking sheet.
3. Roast until the plantain wedges are golden brown, 20 to 30 minutes, tossing halfway through roasting time. Serve warm with Smashed Avocado Butter.

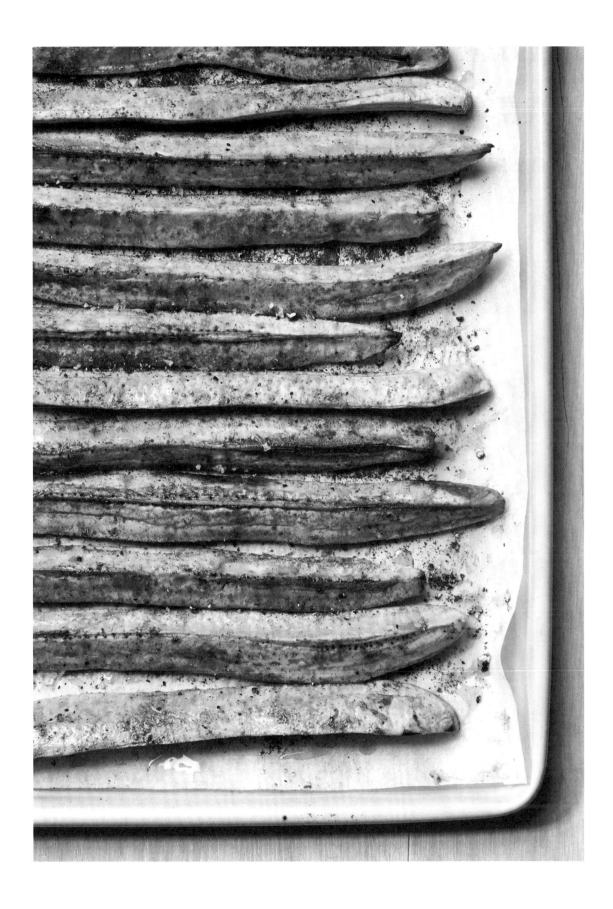

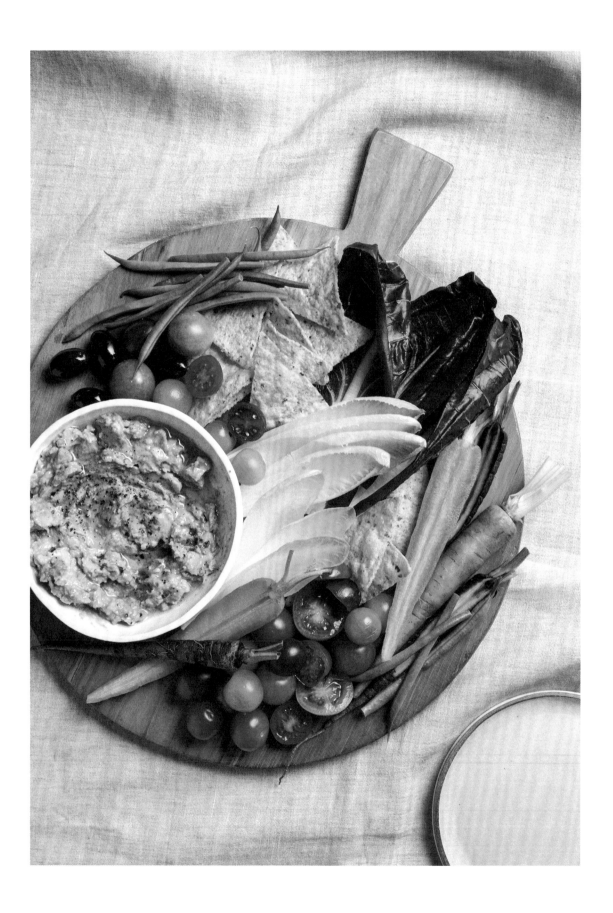

Dairy-Free ◆ Gluten-Free ◆ Grain-Free ◆ Nut-Free
◆ Keto-Friendly ◆ Paleo-Friendly ◆ Vegetarian ◆ *Makes 1 cup (250 mL)*

◆ Smashed Avocado Butter

This fat-fuelled dip is so quick and easy to whip up. I eat it as a work snack or anytime I need a pick-me-up. It's delicious as a dip with Roasted Plantain Wedges (page 204) or spread on Seedy Almond Pulp Crackers (page 192). When I have guests over, I dress it up with crudités, tortilla chips, and olives.

1 avocado, peeled and pitted

1 tablespoon (15 mL) ghee or Plain Jane Ghee (271), at room temperature

1 teaspoon (5 mL) fresh lemon juice

½ teaspoon (2 mL) red chili flakes

Sea salt and black pepper, to taste

Extra-virgin olive oil, to drizzle

1. In a small bowl, smash the avocado with a fork until smooth. Add the ghee, lemon juice, chili flakes, salt, and pepper. Stir to combine. Drizzle with olive oil and enjoy immediately.

Whipped Feta Spread

I first encountered whipped feta at a tapas restaurant in Winnipeg and was instantly obsessed. I immediately went home to learn how to make it, and quickly realized it was as simple as blending feta cheese with some liquid until smooth. I suggest serving it on crostini or Seedy Almond Pulp Crackers (page 192), topped with sliced heirloom tomato and flaky sea salt. For a sweet version, it is excellent topped with chopped pistachios and a drizzle of honey.

Whipped Feta

4 ounces (115 g) sheep's or goat's milk feta cheese

½ cup (125 mL) canned full-fat coconut milk, more as needed

1 teaspoon (5 mL) fresh lemon juice

Crostini or Seedy Almond Pulp Crackers (page 192), to serve

Savoury Toppings

2 heirloom tomatoes, sliced

Flaky sea salt, to taste

Sweet Toppings

½ cup (125 mL) chopped pistachios

1 tablespoon (15 mL) raw liquid honey

1. In a food processor or a high-speed blender, combine the feta cheese, coconut milk, and lemon juice. Process until smooth, 25 to 30 seconds. Add more coconut milk, as needed, to thin the mixture to your desired consistency.

2. Transfer to a serving bowl and top with the savoury or sweet toppings, as desired. Serve with crostini. Store leftover spread in an airtight container in the fridge for up to 1 week.

◆ **Grain-Free and Keto-Friendly:** Serve with Seedy Almond Pulp Crackers instead of crostini.

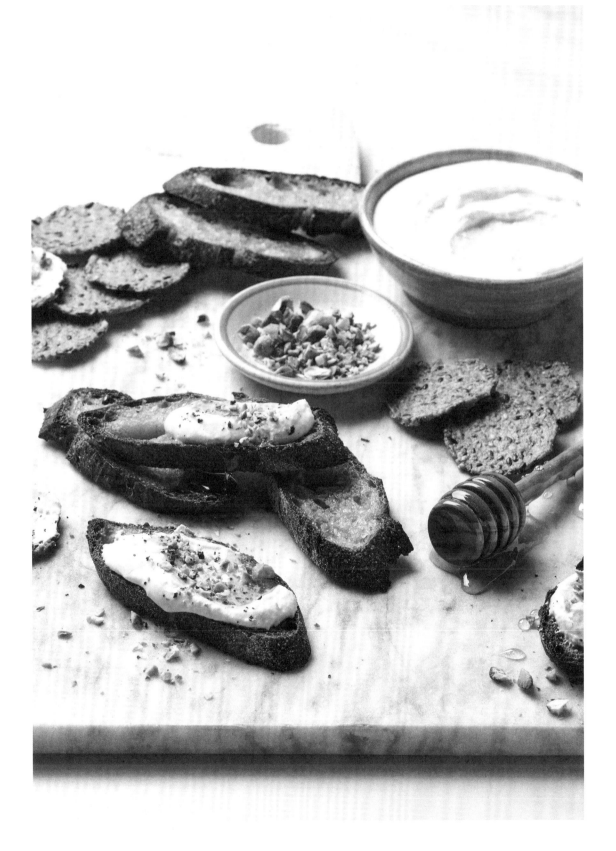

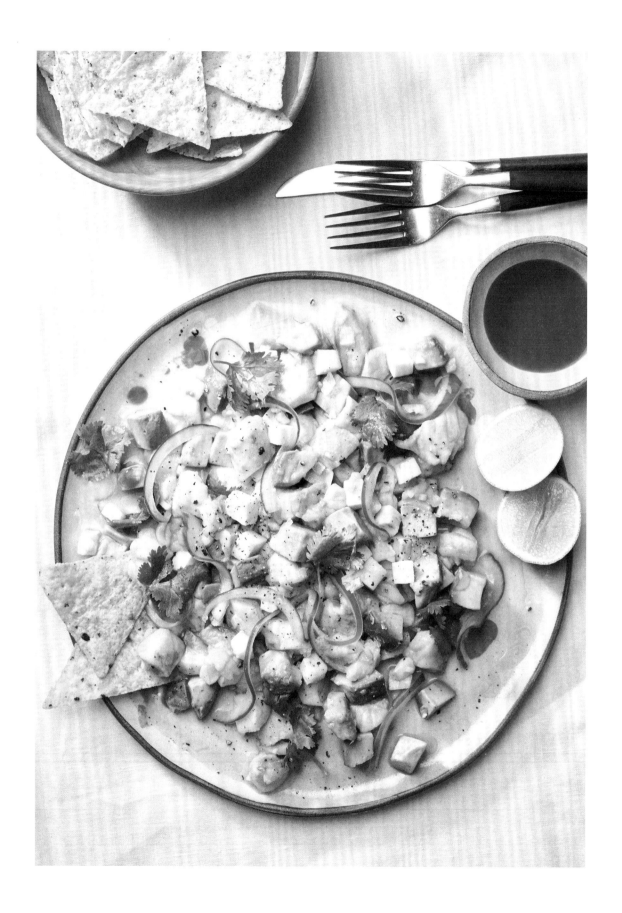

◆ Red Snapper Ceviche

Like salmon, red snapper is high in nourishing omega-3 fatty acids that boost memory and brain function. Although the ceviche is full of good fats and protein, it still feels very light and refreshing—perfect for a hot summer day. When making ceviche, it is crucial to get very high-quality fish, so I suggest buying it from a fishmonger you trust. You can find young coconuts at Asian supermarkets and well-stocked grocery stores.

1 fresh red snapper fillet (about ⅔ pound/300 g), cut into ¾-inch (2 cm) pieces

¼ cup (60 mL) thinly sliced red onion

¼ cup (60 mL) fresh lemon juice

¼ cup (60 mL) fresh lime juice

2 cloves garlic, minced

½ teaspoon (2 mL) sea salt

1 young coconut

2 small avocados, peeled, pitted, and diced

¼ cup (60 mL) loosely packed fresh cilantro leaves

To Serve

Extra-virgin olive oil

Freshly ground black pepper

Tortilla chips or plantain chips

Hot sauce (optional)

1. In a medium bowl, add the snapper, red onion, lemon juice, lime juice, garlic, and salt. Toss to combine. Refrigerate until the fish becomes slightly opaque and firms up a bit, 20 to 25 minutes, stirring the mixture halfway through the chill time.

2. Meanwhile, place the coconut, pointed side up, on a flat surface. Using the heel of a cleaver, firmly hack into the top part of the coconut to break through the shell. Continue hacking until you have a large, square-shaped hole in the shell. Remove the top piece of the shell. Strain the coconut water into a glass. (Now you can drink it!) Using a spoon, scrape out the coconut meat. Chop it into small pieces.

3. Add the coconut meat, avocado, and cilantro to the fish mixture. Stir to combine.

4. To serve, divide the ceviche among plates, drizzle with a bit of olive oil, and sprinkle with pepper. Serve with tortilla chips and hot sauce, if using.

◆ **Grain-Free, Keto-Friendly, and Paleo-Friendly:** Serve with plantain chips instead of tortilla chips.

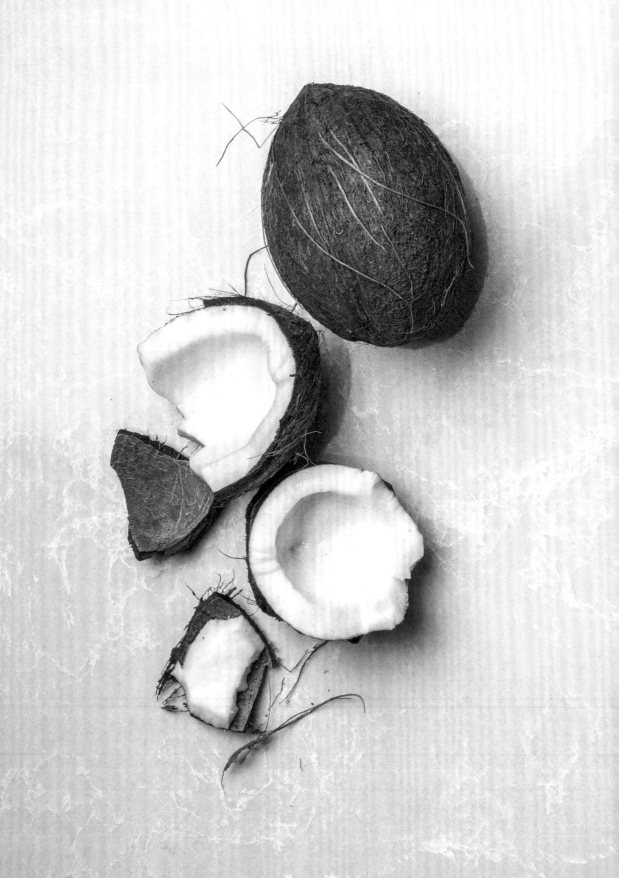

Drinks

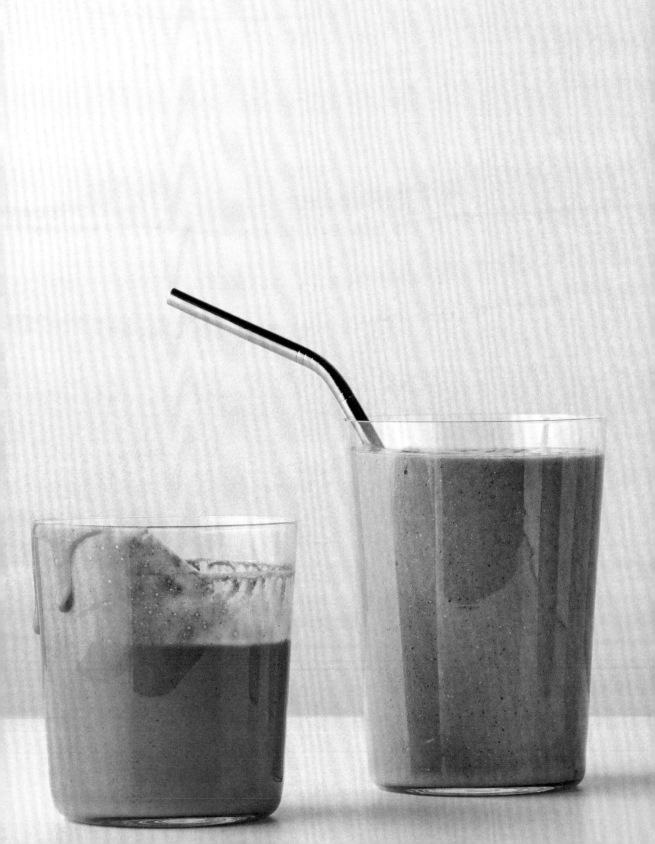

Smoothies
Four Ways

Smoothies are a great way to get extra nutrients into your diet between meals. Most people know to include a lot of fibre-rich fruits and veggies in smoothies, but it's equally important to include healthy fats and protein. This helps keep your blood sugar stable and tides you over to your next meal. In these recipes, I use a variety of protein sources, such as hemp seeds, collagen peptides, and almond butter, but I encourage you to amp up the protein further by adding your favourite protein powder to the mix. Happy blending!

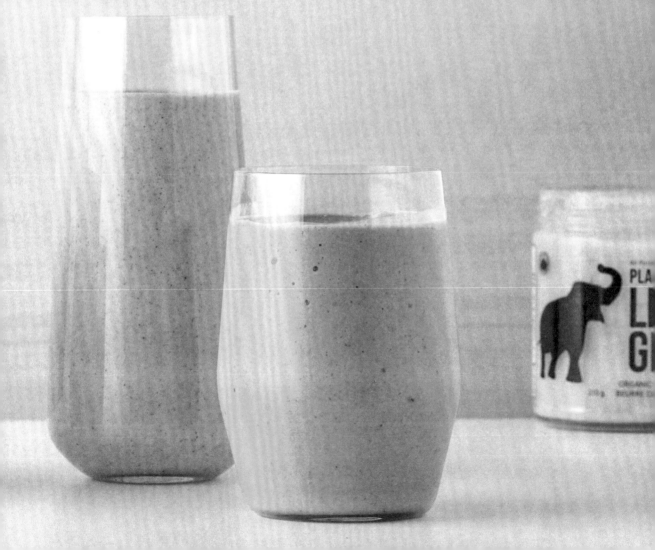

Dairy-Free ◆ Gluten-Free ◆ Grain-Free ◆ Keto-Friendly Option
◆ Paleo-Friendly Option ◆ Vegan ◆ *Serves 1*

Chocolate Olive Oil Smoothie

Who says you can't have chocolate for breakfast? This tasty smoothie is a regular in my morning lineup, and for good reason! It is loaded with nourishing fats from the olive oil, cacao powder, and almond butter. The combination creates a creamy, chocolatey, and energizing elixir that keeps your blood sugar stable and boosts your mood all day long!

1 cup (250 mL) unsweetened almond milk

1 frozen banana

2 tablespoons (30 mL) natural almond butter or Homemade Almond Butter (page 275)

2 tablespoons (30 mL) hemp protein powder (optional)

1½ tablespoons (22 mL) raw cacao powder

1 tablespoon (15 mL) extra-virgin olive oil

Pinch of sea salt

1. In a high-speed blender, combine the almond milk, banana, almond butter, hemp protein powder (if using), cacao powder, olive oil, and salt. Blend on high speed until smooth and creamy, 30 to 60 seconds.
2. Pour into a glass and enjoy immediately.

◆ **Keto-Friendly:** Use ¾ cup (175 mL) frozen cauliflower instead of a frozen banana.
 Paleo-Friendly: Skip the hemp protein powder.

Dairy-Free ◆ Gluten-Free ◆ Grain-Free ◆ Paleo-Friendly ◆ Vegan ◆ *Serves 2*

Tropical Green Smoothie

Green smoothies are one of my favourite ways to start the day! This tropical-inspired green smoothie is so delicious and full of good fats, protein, and fibre to help keep you full until lunchtime. If you have any leftovers, you can pack them in a mason jar to sip on throughout the day. If you use a frozen banana, you may want to add more almond milk to thin the smoothie to your desired consistency.

1½ cups (375 mL) unsweetened almond milk

1 large handful of baby spinach

½ cup (125 mL) packed fresh basil leaves

½ avocado, peeled and pitted

1 cup (250 mL) frozen pineapple chunks

1 banana

1 tablespoon (15 mL) hulled hemp seeds

1. In a high-speed blender, combine the almond milk, spinach, basil, avocado, pineapple, banana, and hemp seeds. Blend on high speed until smooth and creamy, 30 to 60 seconds.
2. Pour into 2 glasses and enjoy immediately.

◆ Pink Collagen Smoothie

This is a delicious pink smoothie that has complete protein, fibre, and healthy fats. Collagen peptides can be found at health food stores and are a key ingredient in this smoothie, helping to promote healthy skin, digestion, and joints. I personally like the sweetness of the frozen banana, but if you are looking to keep your carbohydrate levels down, you can substitute frozen cauliflower.

1 cup (250 mL) unsweetened almond milk

1 cup (250 mL) frozen raspberries

1 frozen banana

⅓ ounce (10 g) scoop of collagen peptides

3 tablespoons (45 mL) natural almond butter or Homemade Almond Butter (page 275)

1 tablespoon (15 mL) hulled hemp seeds

1 teaspoon (5 mL) ghee, Plain Jane Ghee (271), or virgin coconut oil, at room temperature

1. In a high-speed blender, combine the almond milk, raspberries, banana, collagen peptides, almond butter, hemp seeds, and ghee. Blend on high speed until smooth and creamy, 30 to 60 seconds.
2. Pour into a glass and enjoy immediately.

◆ Almond Butter Date Shake

In my early twenties, I worked as a cook at a trendy, plant-based restaurant called *Fresh*. The job was really challenging, so I would order their date almond smoothie for a quick energy boost midday. It worked like a charm! The dates give the smoothie a sweet caramel flavour, which makes it feel like an indulgent treat. My version has extra healthy fats (surprise!), which help slow down the digestion of carbohydrates and keep your blood sugar stable.

1 cup (250 mL) unsweetened almond milk

1 frozen banana

¼ cup (60 mL) natural almond butter or Homemade Almond Butter (page 275)

1 to 2 teaspoons (5 to 10 mL) ghee, Plain Jane Ghee (page 271), or virgin coconut oil, at room temperature

¼ teaspoon (1 mL) cinnamon

¼ teaspoon (1 mL) pure vanilla extract or a pinch of pure vanilla powder

1 soft Medjool date, pitted

Pinch of sea salt

1. In a high-speed blender, combine the almond milk, banana, almond butter, ghee, cinnamon, vanilla, date, and salt. Blend on high speed until smooth and creamy, 30 to 60 seconds.
2. Pour into 2 glasses and enjoy immediately.

◆ **Paleo-Friendly:** Use pure vanilla powder instead of pure vanilla extract.
  Vegan: Use virgin coconut oil instead of ghee.

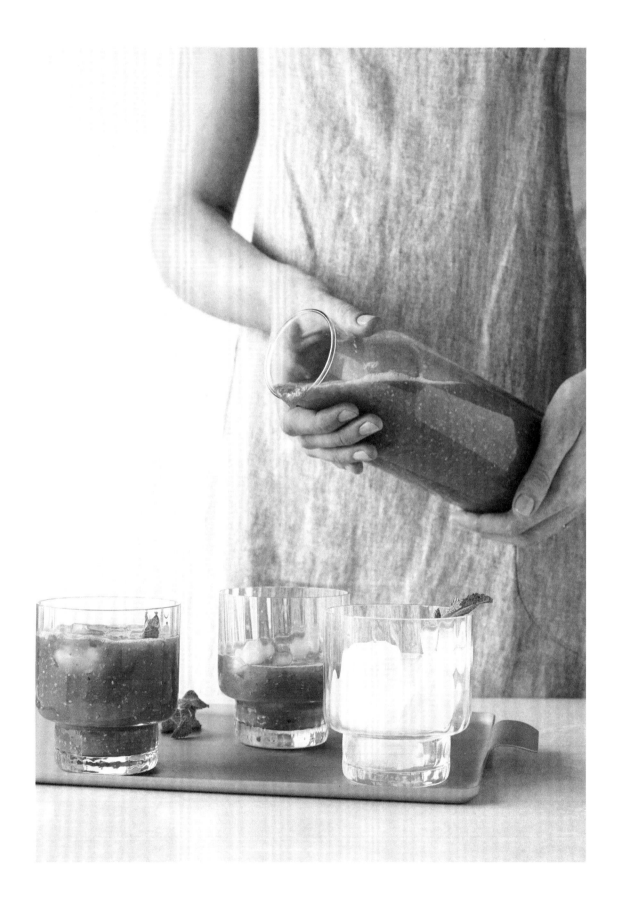

Dairy-Free ◆ Gluten-Free ◆ Grain-Free ◆ Nut-Free
◆ Paleo-Friendly ◆ Vegan Option ◆ Vegetarian ◆ *Serves 6*

◆ Watermelon Chia Fresca

This fun version of agua fresca is perfect for cooling off at a summer barbecue or picnic. Chia seeds are small but mighty—they add a healthy dose of protein and good fats to this refreshing summer drink. I love how simple it is to whip up. Just soak the chia seeds and blend them with some fresh watermelon, lime juice, and a touch of honey. Whoosh, your favourite summer drink is ready to serve!

3 tablespoons (45 mL) white chia seeds

1 cup (250 mL) water

4 cups (1 L) chopped seedless watermelon

3 tablespoons (45 mL) fresh lime juice

Zest of 1 lime

2 tablespoons (30 mL) raw liquid honey

Fresh mint leaves, for garnish (optional)

1. In a small bowl, add the chia seeds and water. Soak the chia seeds until the mixture becomes gelatinous, about 10 minutes.
2. In a blender, combine the watermelon, lime juice, lime zest, and honey. Blend on high speed until smooth, about 30 seconds.
3. Add the chia seeds to the blender and pulse to combine.
4. Chill in the refrigerator. Pour into glasses and garnish with mint leaves, if desired.

◆ **Vegan:** Use pure maple syrup instead of honey.

Buttered Tahini Cardamom Latte

I did not know that it was possible to love tahini any more than I already do, but this tahini latte sure proved me wrong! Tahini adds an irresistible nutty flavour to this energizing butter coffee. If you drink a cup first thing in the morning, it will give you a boost of stable energy without a caffeine crash. I haven't added any sweetener to the recipe, but feel free to sweeten to taste.

1½ cups (375 mL) hot brewed coffee

1 tablespoon (15 mL) tahini

1 teaspoon (5 mL) ghee or Plain Jane Ghee (page 271)

Pinch of ground cardamom

⅓ ounce (10 g) scoop of collagen peptides (optional)

1. In a blender, combine the coffee, tahini, ghee, cardamom, and collagen peptides, if using. Blend on high speed until frothy and creamy, about 30 seconds.

2. Pour into a mug and enjoy immediately.

◆ **Vegetarian:** Skip the collagen peptides.

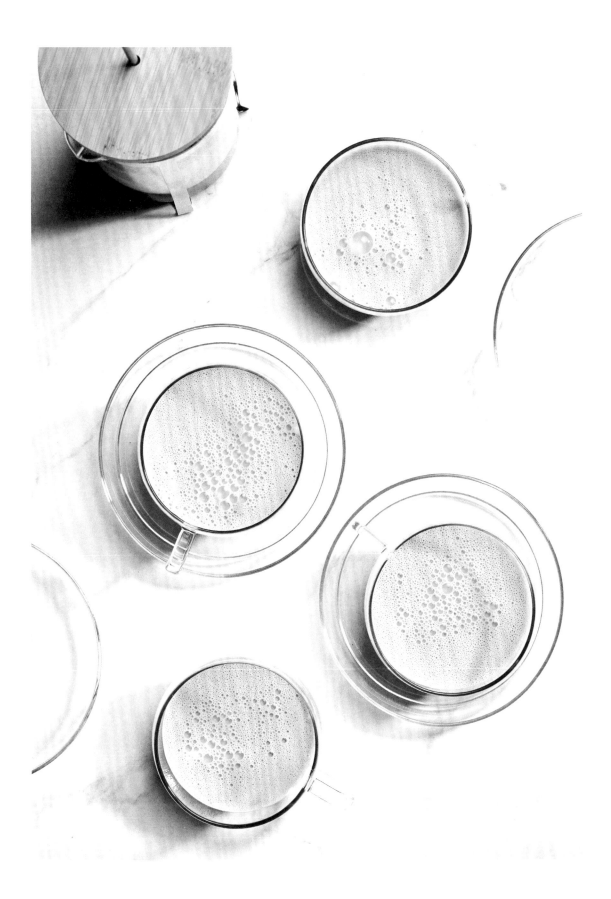

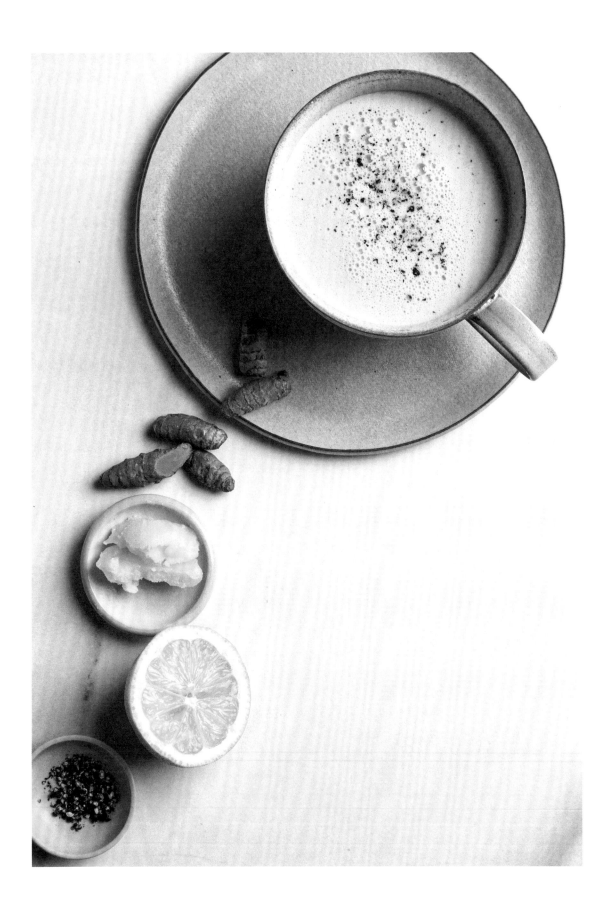

◆ Bone Broth Turmeric Latte

If a turmeric latte and bone broth got married, this would be their baby! This warming and soothing beverage is full of gut-loving benefits from bone broth, ghee, and turmeric. Bone broth is a fantastic source of collagen protein, ghee is rich in butyric acid (a short-chain fatty acid that nourishes the cells of the intestines), and turmeric is an anti-inflammatory. Together, they are a powerhouse for your digestion.

1½ cups (375 mL) Chicken or Beef Bone Broth (page 272)

1½ teaspoons (7 mL) ghee or Plain Jane Ghee (page 271)

½ teaspoon (2 mL) ground turmeric

½ teaspoon (2 mL) fresh lemon juice

Pinch of black pepper

1. In a small saucepan over medium heat, bring the bone broth to a simmer.
2. Pour the bone broth into a blender. Add the ghee, turmeric, lemon juice, and pepper. Blend on high speed until frothy and creamy, about 30 seconds.
3. Pour into a mug and enjoy immediately.

Pink Chai Latte

Inspired by my best-selling Pink Chai tea blend, I created this version you can make at home with fresh ingredients (available at a health food store). Tulsi is a caffeine-free herb known for its calming properties, which makes it the perfect tea to have before bed. The tea is brewed on the stove until the spices are infused, then strained and blended with coconut butter until frothy. To make an iced Pink Chai Latte, simply pour the blended drink over ice.

8 cardamom pods

1 cinnamon stick

5 black peppercorns

¼ teaspoon (1 mL) fennel seeds

2 whole cloves

1 (2-inch/5 cm) piece of fresh organic ginger, peeled and grated

2 teaspoons (10 mL) peeled, grated organic red beet (1 small beet)

2 tablespoons (30 mL) loose leaf tulsi tea

2½ cups (625 mL) unsweetened almond milk

2 teaspoons (10 mL) coconut butter or virgin coconut oil

Raw liquid honey, to taste (optional)

1. Using a mortar and pestle (or the flat edge of a heavy knife), crush the cardamom, cinnamon, peppercorns, fennel seeds, and cloves.

2. In a medium saucepan, add the crushed spices, grated ginger, grated beetroot, tea leaves, and almond milk. Stir to combine. Bring to a boil and then remove from the heat. Cover and let steep for 7 minutes.

3. Using a fine mesh strainer, strain the tea into a blender. Add the coconut butter. Blend on high speed until frothy and creamy, about 30 seconds. Add the honey to sweeten to taste, if using.

4. Pour into 2 mugs and enjoy immediately.

◆ **Vegan:** Skip the raw honey.

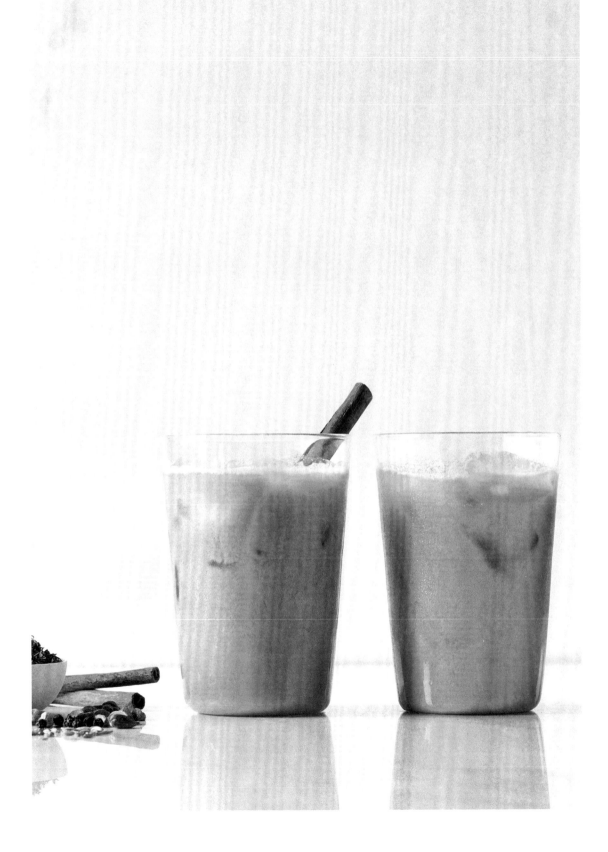

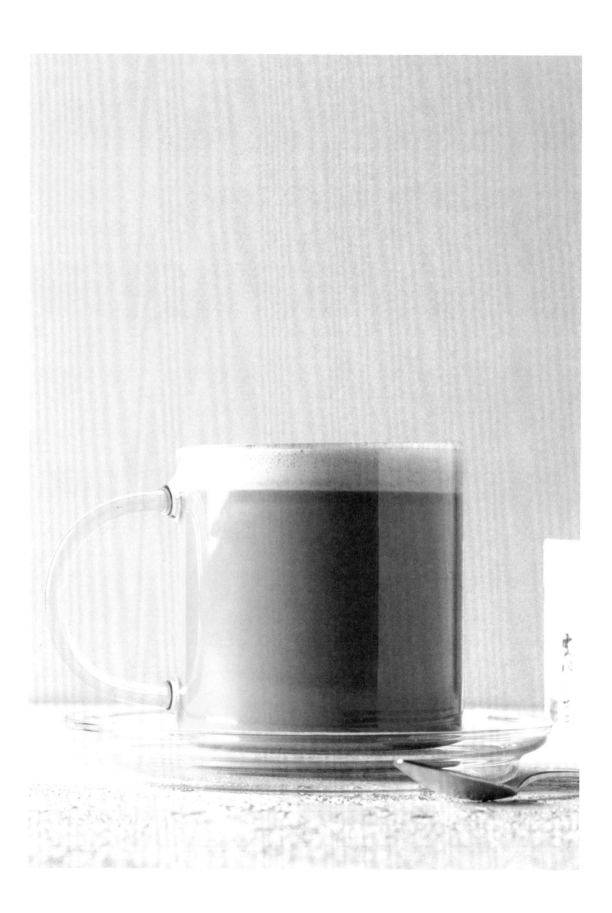

Dairy-Free ◆ Gluten-Free ◆ Grain-Free ◆ Nut-Free
◆ Keto-Friendly ◆ Paleo-Friendly ◆ Vegetarian Option ◆ *Serves 1*

◆ I Love You So Matcha

These days, coffee is fuelling my busy mornings, but now and then I like to switch it up with a fat-fuelled matcha latte. I like Ippodo Tea matcha, as it is very smooth and balanced, so you don't need to add any sweetener. Adding a scoop of collagen peptides gives the latte extra staying power and beautifying benefits that help you glow from the inside out. To make an iced matcha latte, simply pour the blended drink over ice.

1 cup (250 mL) boiling water

1 teaspoon (5 mL) matcha powder

1 teaspoon (5 mL) coconut butter or virgin coconut oil

1 teaspoon (5 mL) ghee or Plain Jane Ghee (page 271)

⅓ ounce (10 g) scoop of collagen peptides (optional)

Pinch of cinnamon

1. Pour the boiling water into a mug and let it sit for 30 seconds to cool slightly.
2. Transfer the water to a blender. Add the matcha powder, coconut butter, ghee, collagen peptides (if using), and cinnamon. Blend on high speed until frothy and creamy, about 30 seconds.
3. Pour back into the mug and enjoy immediately.

◆ **Vegetarian:** Skip the collagen peptides.

◆ Cacao Butter Hot Chocolate

This hot chocolate is frothy, creamy, and lightly sweetened—the perfect thing to cuddle up with on a cold winter day. Cacao butter is a natural fat that is derived from cacao beans. Its subtle chocolate flavour and creaminess make it the perfect addition to a steaming cup of hot chocolate goodness.

1½ cups (375 mL) unsweetened almond milk

2 tablespoons (30 mL) cacao powder

2 tablespoons (30 mL) cacao butter, chopped

1 teaspoon (5 mL) pure maple syrup, more to taste

½ teaspoon (2 mL) pure vanilla extract or ¼ teaspoon (1 mL) pure vanilla powder

Pinch of sea salt

1. In a small saucepan over medium heat, bring the almond milk to a simmer.
2. Pour the almond milk into a blender. Add the cacao powder, cacao butter, maple syrup, vanilla, and salt. Blend on high speed until frothy, smooth, and creamy, 30 to 60 seconds. Add more maple syrup, to taste.
3. Pour into a mug and enjoy immediately.

◆ **Keto-Friendly:** Skip the maple syrup.
Paleo-Friendly: Use pure vanilla powder instead of pure vanilla extract.

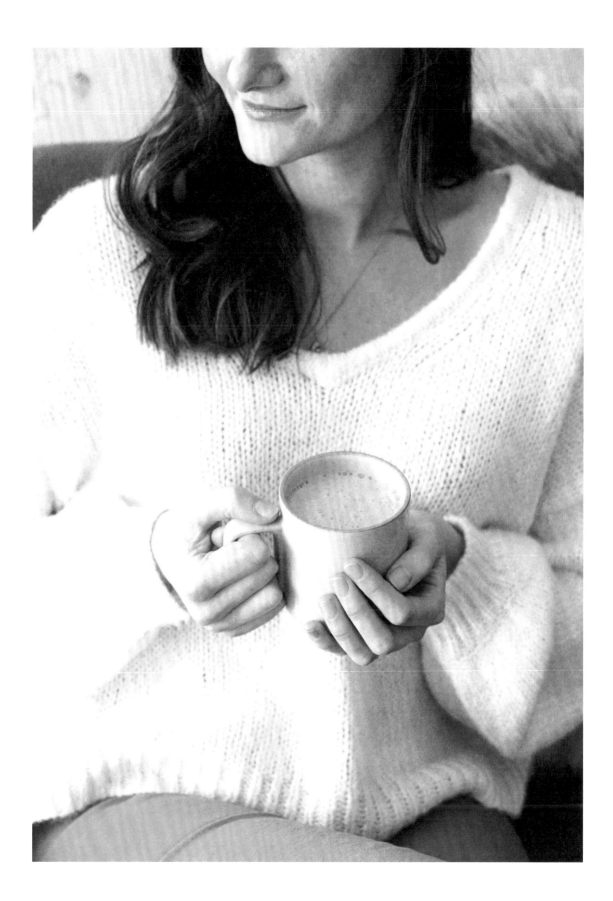

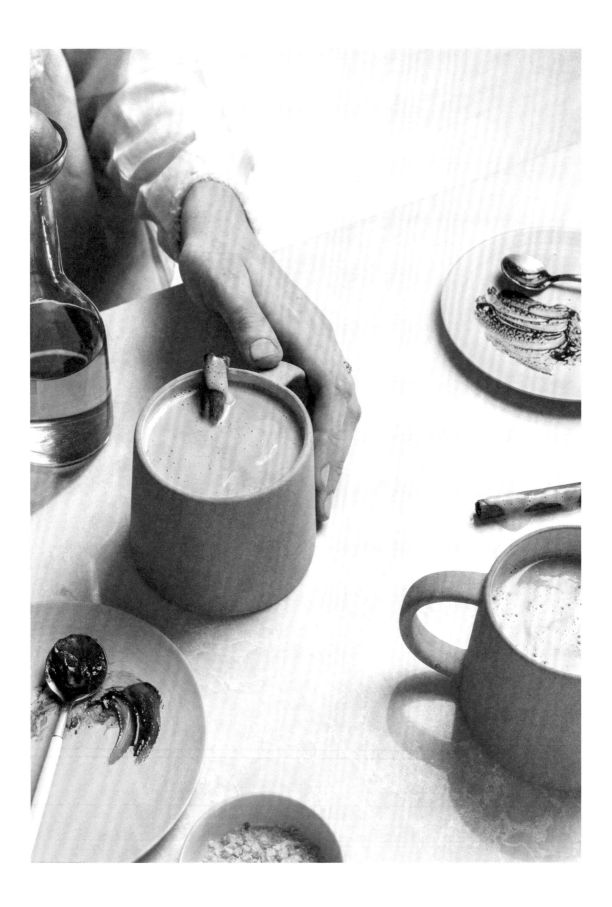

Dairy-Free ◆ Gluten-Free ◆ Grain-Free ◆ Nut-Free ◆ Vegetarian ◆ *Serves 4*

◆ Hot Buttered Cider

One year, the lovely folks at Evergreen Brick Works, a local farmers market, developed this spiked winter cocktail using my ghee for their menu. It has a sweet and spiced flavour that is perfect for cozying up in the fall. If you don't have spiced whiskey in your liquor cabinet, you can substitute spiced rum instead.

3 cups (750 mL) apple cider

2 tablespoons (30 mL) water

1½ teaspoons (7 mL) ghee or Plain Jane Ghee (page 271)

½ teaspoon (2 mL) pure vanilla extract

Pinch of smoked sea salt

4 ounces (115 mL) spiced whiskey

4 cinnamon sticks, to serve

1. In a small saucepan over medium heat, bring the apple cider to a simmer.

2. Pour the warmed cider into a blender. Add the water, ghee, vanilla, and smoked salt. Blend on high speed until frothy and creamy, about 30 seconds.

3. Pour into mugs. Add 1 ounce (30 mL) spiced whiskey to each mug. Add a cinnamon stick to each mug and stir to combine. Enjoy immediately.

◆ Mango Cardamom Lassi

This refreshing drink saved me during a major heat wave in Toronto. The coconut yogurt base is cooling and refreshing, perfect for those sweltering days. I like to buy Indian mangoes when they are in season in the summer, but any ripe and juicy mangoes will do the trick. To make mango lassi popsicles, leave out the ice and freeze the mixture in an ice-pop mould for at least 4 hours.

1 cup (250 mL) chopped fresh mango

⅔ cup (150 mL) plain coconut yogurt or plain full-fat yogurt

2 tablespoons (30 mL) fresh lime juice

2 tablespoons (30 mL) pure maple syrup

Pinch of ground cardamom

Pinch of sea salt

5 ice cubes

1. In a high-speed blender, combine the mango, coconut yogurt, lime juice, maple syrup, cardamom, salt, and ice cubes. Blend on high speed until smooth, about 30 seconds.
2. Pour into 2 glasses and enjoy immediately.

◆ **Vegan:** Use coconut yogurt.

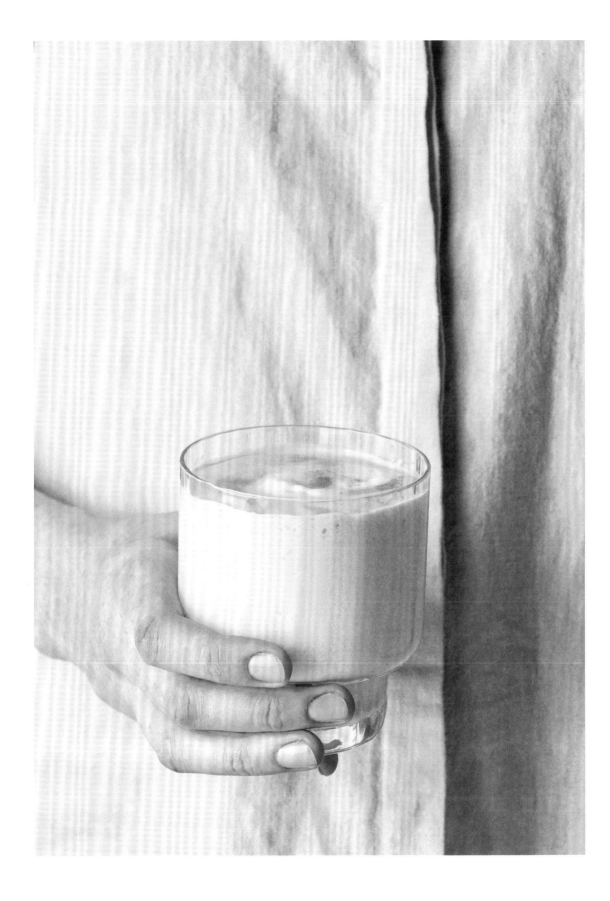

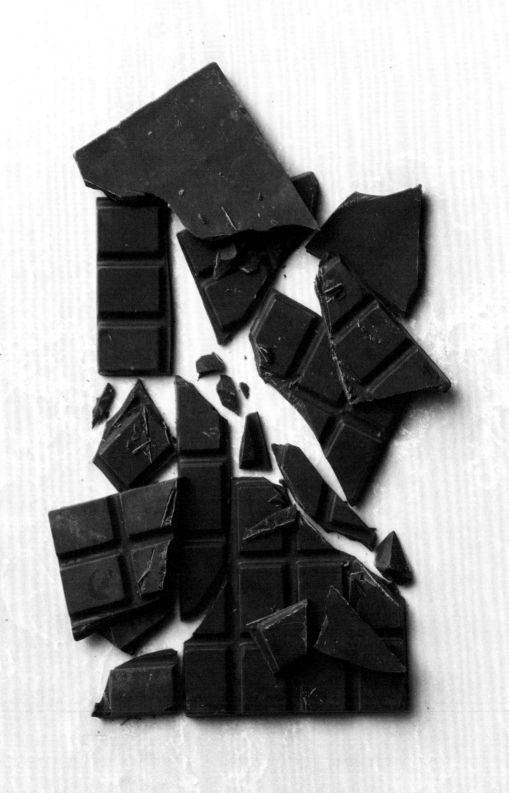

Desserts

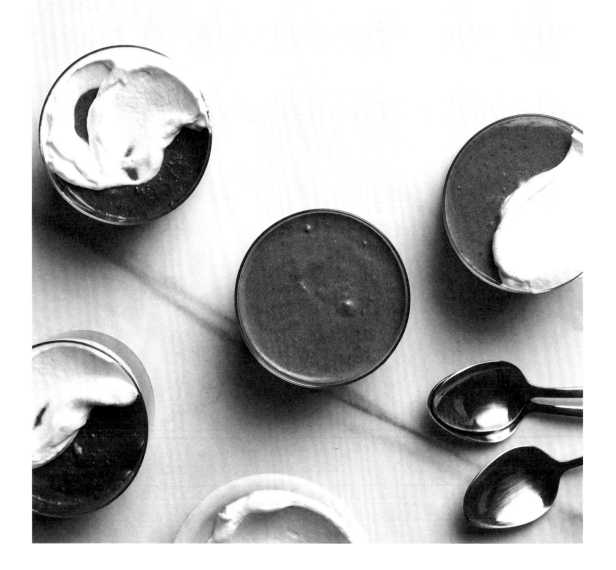

◆ Chocolate Chia Mousse

This chocolate chia mousse is a great dessert to serve on a special occasion. It is creamy, satisfying, and super easy to make. It's also full of healthy fats from coconut milk, chia seeds, and almond butter. This mousse is quite filling, so you only need a small portion to satisfy those chocolate cravings.

2 cans (14 ounces/400 mL each) full-fat coconut milk

2 teaspoons (10 mL) black chia seeds

8 soft Medjool dates, pitted

¼ cup (60 mL) raw cacao powder

2 tablespoons (30 mL) pure maple syrup

2 tablespoons (30 mL) natural almond butter or Homemade Almond Butter (page 275)

½ teaspoon (2 mL) pure vanilla extract or ¼ teaspoon (1 mL) pure vanilla powder

Pinch of sea salt

Coconut Whipped Cream (page 274), to serve (optional)

1. In a food processor or a high-speed blender, combine the coconut milk, chia seeds, dates, cacao powder, almond butter, vanilla, and salt. Blend on high speed, scraping down the sides as needed, until smooth, 20 to 30 seconds.

2. Divide the mixture into 4 glasses or serving bowls. Refrigerate for 30 minutes to set.

3. Just before serving, top with Coconut Whipped Cream, if desired.

◆ **Paleo-Friendly:** Use pure vanilla powder instead of pure vanilla extract.

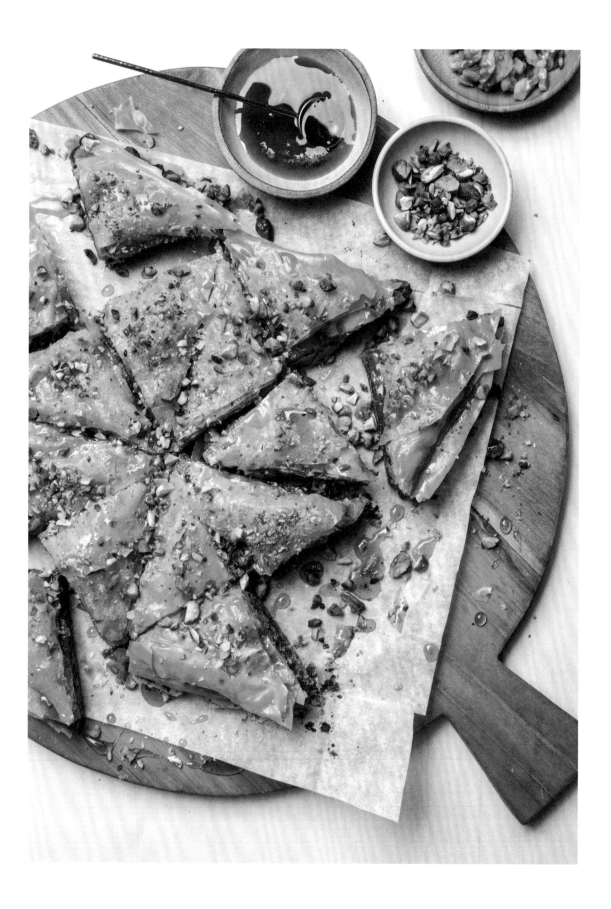

◆ Maple Pistachio Baklava

If I had to pick a favourite dessert, it would be baklava. Unfortunately, store-bought baklava is full of refined sugar and unhealthy oils, so I created this recipe, which is lightly sweetened with maple syrup and uses ghee. Be sure to check the ingredients in the phyllo pastry to ensure that it is pure butter pastry, which does not contain harmful vegetable oils or trans fats.

½ cup (125 mL) ghee or Plain Jane Ghee (page 271), melted

1 cup (250 mL) raw walnuts

1 cup (250 mL) + 2 tablespoons (30 mL) raw shelled pistachios, divided

¼ cup (60 mL) coconut sugar

1 teaspoon (5 mL) cinnamon

½ teaspoon (2 mL) ground cardamom

16 ounces (450 g) all-butter phyllo pastry, defrosted according to package directions

¼ cup (60 mL) pure maple syrup

1. Position a rack in the middle of the oven. Preheat the oven to 350°F (180°C). Line the bottom of a glass 8-inch (2 L) square baking dish with parchment paper. Lightly brush the parchment paper with some of the melted ghee.

2. In a food processor, combine the walnuts and 1 cup (250 mL) of the pistachios. Pulse several times until the nuts are roughly chopped. Transfer to a medium bowl and add the coconut sugar, cinnamon, and cardamom. Stir to combine.

3. Using scissors, cut the sheets of phyllo pastry into 8-inch (20 cm) squares. You'll need 20 squares of pastry. Place one square sheet in the bottom of the baking dish.

4. Lightly brush some ghee over the pastry and place another sheet of phyllo on top. Repeat until you have 8 sheets of pastry layered and brushed with ghee.

5. Add half of the nut mixture on top and spread it evenly across the pastry. Add 4 more sheets of pastry, brushing ghee on each sheet before adding another layer.

6. Add the remaining nut mixture on top and spread it evenly across the pastry.

7. Add 8 more sheets of phyllo pastry, brushing ghee on each sheet before adding another layer. Brush ghee on the final sheet of pastry. Using a sharp knife, carefully slice the baklava into 8 triangles. To make smaller pieces, slice each triangle in half. Bake for 30 to 35 minutes, rotating the dish once after 15 minutes, until the pastry is golden brown and crispy. Remove from the oven and let cool for 30 minutes.

8. In a small bowl, stir together the maple syrup and the remaining melted ghee. Pour the mixture over the surface of the baklava, letting it sink into the cracks and soak the pastry.

9. Finely chop the remaining 2 tablespoons (30 mL) pistachios. Sprinkle them over the baklava. Let sit for at least 1 hour before serving to allow the liquid to soak in. Store the baklava in an airtight container at room temperature for up to 3 weeks.

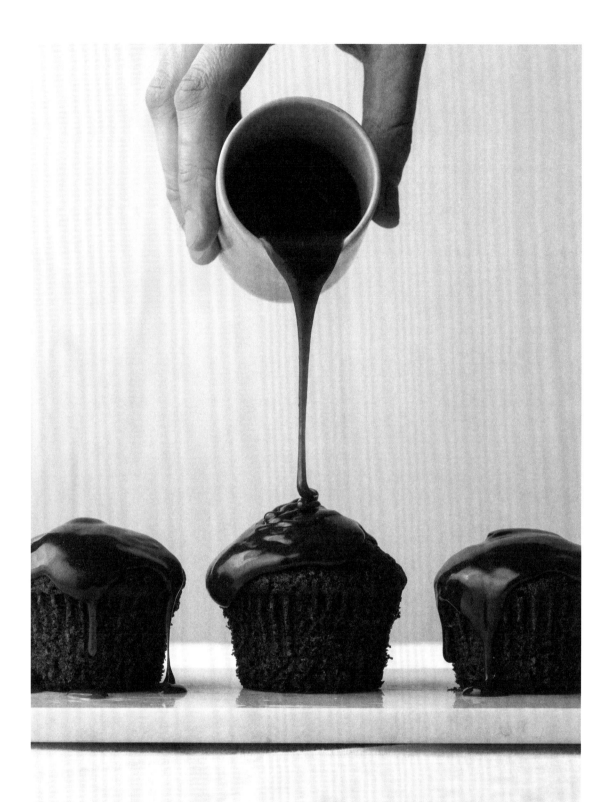

◆ Kabocha Squash Cupcakes with Dulce de Coco

My three-year-old niece is obsessed with these cupcakes! They are super light and fluffy, thanks to a good dose of olive oil. I make them in the fall when squash is in season, and they taste just like pumpkin spice! Cassava flour is a gluten-free, grain-free flour. If you don't have cassava flour, you can substitute gluten-free all-purpose flour or sprouted or light spelt flour. The squash can be roasted in advance to cut down on prep time. To give the dulce de coco a caramel-like texture, you will need to use coconut milk that does not contain any gums or thickeners. Aroy-D is a brand I like that contains only coconut extract and water.

Kabocha Squash Cupcakes

1 small kabocha or buttercup squash, cut in half and seeded

1 tablespoon (15 mL) avocado oil

1 cup (250 mL) extra-virgin olive oil

3 pasture-raised or organic eggs

½ teaspoon (2 mL) pure vanilla extract or ¼ teaspoon (1 mL) pure vanilla powder

1½ cups (375 mL) cassava flour

1¼ cups (300 mL) coconut sugar

1½ teaspoons (7 mL) baking powder

1½ teaspoons (7 mL) cinnamon

½ teaspoon (2 mL) baking soda

½ teaspoon (2 mL) ground cardamom

½ teaspoon (2 mL) ground ginger

Pinch of ground cloves

½ teaspoon (2 mL) sea salt

Dulce de Coco

1 can (14 ounces/400 mL) full-fat coconut milk

½ cup (125 mL) coconut sugar

½ teaspoon (2 mL) sea salt

1 tablespoon (15 mL) ghee or Plain Jane Ghee (page 271), at room temperature

½ teaspoon (2 mL) pure vanilla extract or ¼ teaspoon (1 mL) pure vanilla powder

1. Preheat the oven to 400°F (200°C). Line 12 muffin cups with paper liners (unless you are using a silicone muffin tray).

2. **Make the Kabocha Squash Cupcakes** In a large bowl, coat the squash with avocado oil. Place it, cut side down, on an unlined baking sheet. Roast until the squash is fork-tender, 30 to 35 minutes. Scoop out the flesh of half the squash and reserve the other half for another use.

3. Lower the oven temperature to 325°F (160°C).

4. In a blender or a food processor, add the squash flesh. Blend until smooth, 10 to 15 seconds.

5. In a large bowl, add 1 cup (250 mL) of the squash purée, olive oil, eggs, and vanilla. Whisk to combine.

6. In a medium bowl, combine the cassava flour, coconut sugar, baking powder, cinnamon, baking soda, cardamom, ginger, cloves, and salt. Add the flour mixture to the squash mixture and whisk to incorporate.

7. Spoon the batter into the prepared muffin cups (or directly into silicone muffin cups), filling each about two-thirds full. Bake until a toothpick inserted in the centre of a muffin comes out clean, 20 to 25 minutes. Let cool for 10 to 15 minutes.

recipe continues

recipe continued

8. **Meanwhile, Make the Dulce de Coco** In a large skillet (not a saucepan) over medium-high heat, bring the coconut milk to a boil, then reduce the heat to medium. Stir in the coconut sugar and salt. Simmer, stirring constantly, until the mixture thickens to a caramel-like consistency, 8 to 10 minutes. Remove from the heat. Stir in the ghee and vanilla.

9. To serve, remove the cupcakes from the paper liners and place them on a serving dish. Drizzle the Dulce de Coco over the cupcakes, letting it drip down the sides. Store leftover cupcakes, covered, at room temperature for up to 2 days.

◆ **Paleo-Friendly:** Use pure vanilla powder instead of pure vanilla extract.

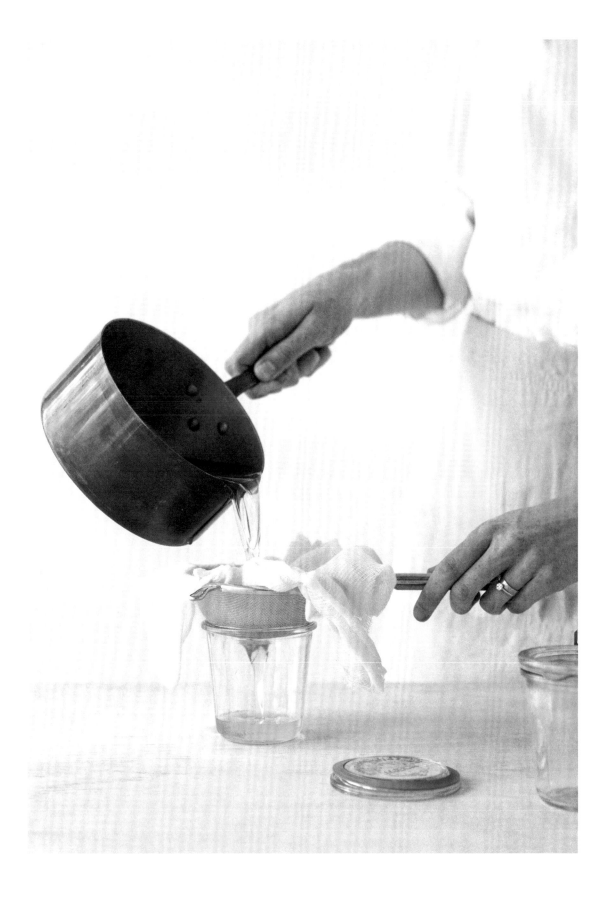

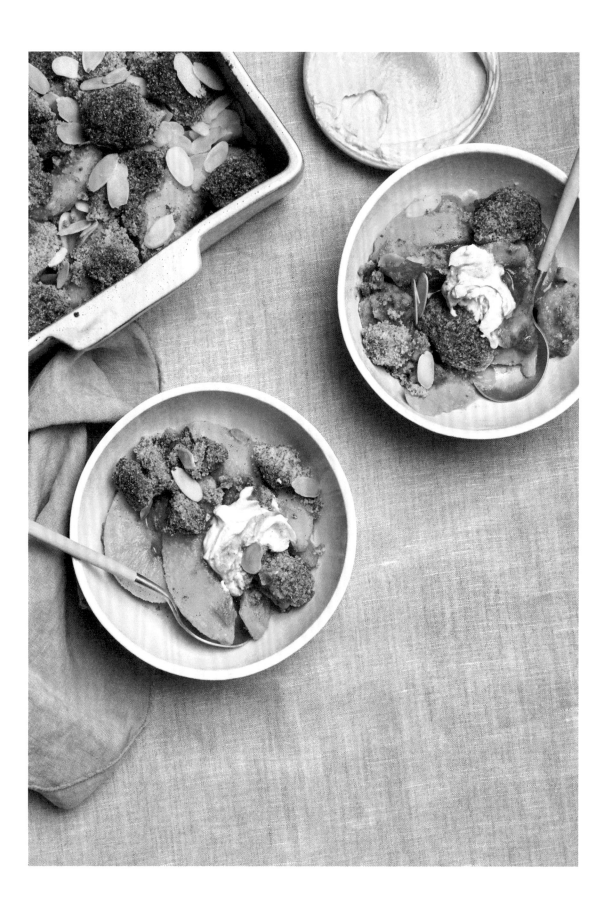

Grain-Free Peach Almond Crumble

This crumble is a melt-in-your-mouth combination of caramelized, juicy peaches topped with large pebbles of buttery almond shortbread. I make this dessert in the summer when peaches are really soft and ripe, but you can substitute berries when peaches are not in season. The great thing is that this dessert is gluten-free and grain-free, meaning that just about anyone can enjoy it!

Peach Filling

2 pounds (900 g) firm-ripe peaches, peeled, pitted, and thinly sliced (5 to 6 peaches)

⅓ cup (75 mL) pure maple syrup

3 tablespoons (45 mL) arrowroot starch

½ teaspoon (2 mL) cinnamon

¼ teaspoon (1 mL) cardamom

½ teaspoon (2 mL) sea salt

Almond Crumble Topping

1 cup (250 mL) super-fine blanched almond flour

½ cup (125 mL) coconut flour

½ cup (125 mL) coconut sugar

¼ teaspoon (1 mL) sea salt

7 tablespoons (105 mL) ghee or Plain Jane Ghee (page 271), at room temperature

¼ cup (60 mL) sliced raw almonds

Coconut Whipped Cream (page 274) or coconut ice cream, to serve

1. Preheat the oven to 325°F (160°C).

2. **Make the Peach Filling** In a large bowl, mix together the peaches, maple syrup, arrowroot starch, cinnamon, cardamom, and salt. Transfer to a glass 8-inch (2 L) square baking dish and spread out the mixture evenly.

3. **Make the Almond Crumble Topping** In another large bowl, combine the almond flour, coconut flour, coconut sugar, and salt. Add the ghee and stir to combine. Using your hands, squeeze the flour mixture together to form small, pebble-like pieces, about ½ inch to ¾ inch (1 to 2 cm) in size.

4. Scatter the pieces of almond crumble evenly over the filling. The crumble pieces should be lightly touching each other and covering most of the surface. Sprinkle the sliced almonds over the crumble pieces. Bake until the filling bubbles up at the sides, 30 to 35 minutes.

5. Set the oven to broil. Broil until the sliced almonds and crumble topping turn golden brown, 2 to 3 minutes. Remove from the oven and let sit for 10 to 15 minutes. Serve warm with Coconut Whipped Cream. Store leftover crumble, covered, in the fridge for up to 1 week.

Grain-Free Blackberry Clafoutis

One of my regular customers at the farmers market created this clafoutis using my ghee. Originally there wasn't any sweetness apart from the fruit, but I've added a touch of maple syrup to lightly sweeten the recipe. This clafoutis is very quick to make, as the batter is made in a blender and then simply poured over the fruit before baking. The great thing is that you can use whatever fruit you have on hand. I use blackberries when they are in season, but raspberries or cherries are excellent options, too.

1 cup (250 mL) fresh blackberries

2 tablespoons (30 mL) ghee or Plain Jane Ghee (page 271), more for the pie plate, at room temperature

½ cup (125 mL) arrowroot starch

2 tablespoons (30 mL) coconut flour

1 cup (250 mL) canned full-fat coconut milk

4 pasture-raised or organic eggs

2 tablespoons (30 mL) pure maple syrup

1 tablespoon (15 mL) pure vanilla extract or 1½ teaspoons (7 mL) pure vanilla powder

¼ teaspoon (1 mL) sea salt

1 teaspoon (5 mL) coconut milk powder, to serve (optional)

1. Preheat the oven to 325°F (160°C). Grease a 9-inch (23 cm) pie plate with ghee.

2. Arrange the blackberries in a single layer on the surface of the pie plate.

3. In a blender or a food processor, combine the ghee, arrowroot starch, coconut flour, coconut milk, eggs, maple syrup, vanilla, and salt. Blend until smooth, 15 to 20 seconds.

4. Pour the batter over the blackberries. Bake until the top of the clafoutis is golden brown and puffed up, 40 to 50 minutes. Remove from the oven and let cool for 15 minutes.

5. Using a fine mesh strainer, dust the cake with coconut milk powder, if using.

6. To serve, scoop the clafoutis onto plates with a large spoon. Store leftover clafoutis, covered, in the fridge for up to 1 week.

◆ **Keto-Friendly:** Skip the maple syrup. Use vanilla powder instead of pure vanilla extract.

Paleo-Friendly: Use pure vanilla powder instead of pure vanilla extract.

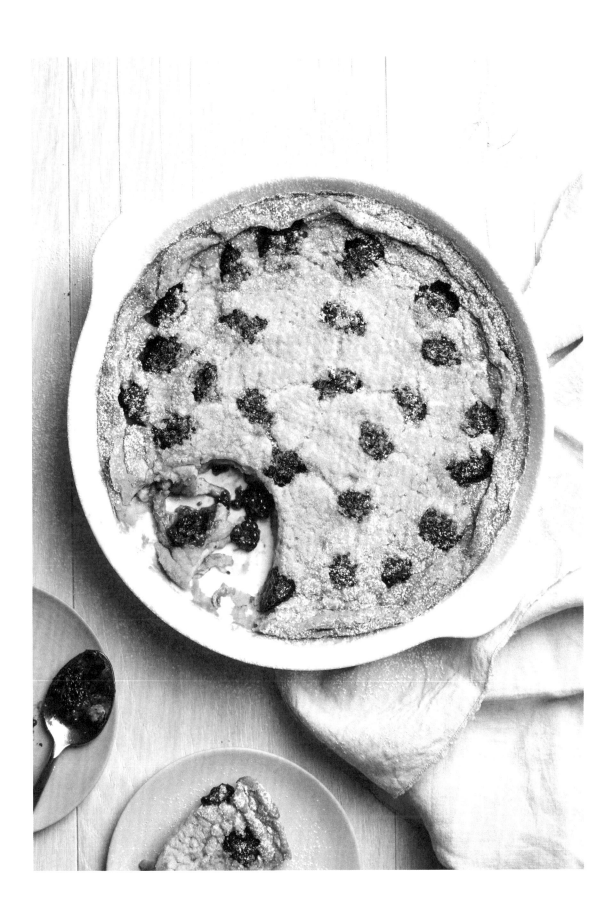

Fudgy Tahini Blondies with Walnuts

These blondies are crinkly on the outside, fudgy on the inside, and have a crunch of toasted walnuts in every bite. As if that were not enough, the ghee, tahini, and coconut sugar combine to give the blondies a caramel flavour that is totally out of this world. If you can get your hands on some brown butter ghee, it will add a nutty flavour that takes these treats to the next level!

½ cup (125 mL) raw walnuts

1½ cups (375 mL) coconut sugar

½ cup (125 mL) ghee or Plain Jane Ghee (page 271), at room temperature

¼ cup (60 mL) tahini

2 pasture-raised or organic eggs

2 teaspoons (10 mL) pure vanilla extract or 1 teaspoon (5 mL) pure vanilla powder

1 cup (250 mL) packed sprouted or light spelt flour or cassava flour

½ teaspoon (2 mL) baking powder

¼ teaspoon (1 mL) sea salt

Flaky sea salt, to serve (optional)

1. Preheat the oven to 350°F (180°C). Line the bottom of a glass 8-inch (2 L) square baking dish with parchment paper.

2. Heat a dry, large skillet over medium-high heat. Add the walnuts in a single layer. Toast for 5 to 6 minutes, tossing occasionally, until the walnuts are fragrant and browned. Transfer to a cutting board to cool. Roughly chop into pieces.

3. In a large bowl, using a wooden spoon, cream together the coconut sugar and ghee. Add the tahini, eggs, and vanilla. Stir to combine.

4. Add the spelt flour, baking powder, and salt. Stir until just incorporated, then fold in the walnut pieces. Transfer the batter to the prepared baking dish, using a spatula to smooth it out evenly.

5. Bake until the centre is just firm to the touch, 25 to 30 minutes. You want the blondies to be slightly underbaked, so that they are still very moist and fudgy on the inside. Remove from the oven and sprinkle immediately with flaky sea salt, if using. Let cool for 30 minutes, then slice into squares. Store leftover blondies, covered, at room temperature for up to 1 week.

◆ **Gluten-Free:** Use gluten-free all-purpose flour instead of sprouted or light spelt flour.
Paleo-Friendly: Use pure vanilla powder instead of pure vanilla extract. Use cassava flour instead of light spelt flour.

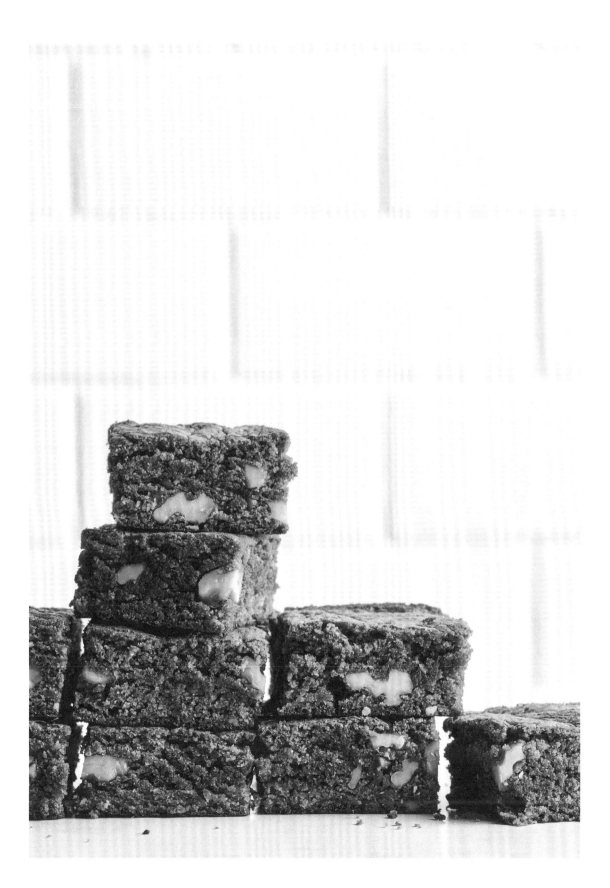

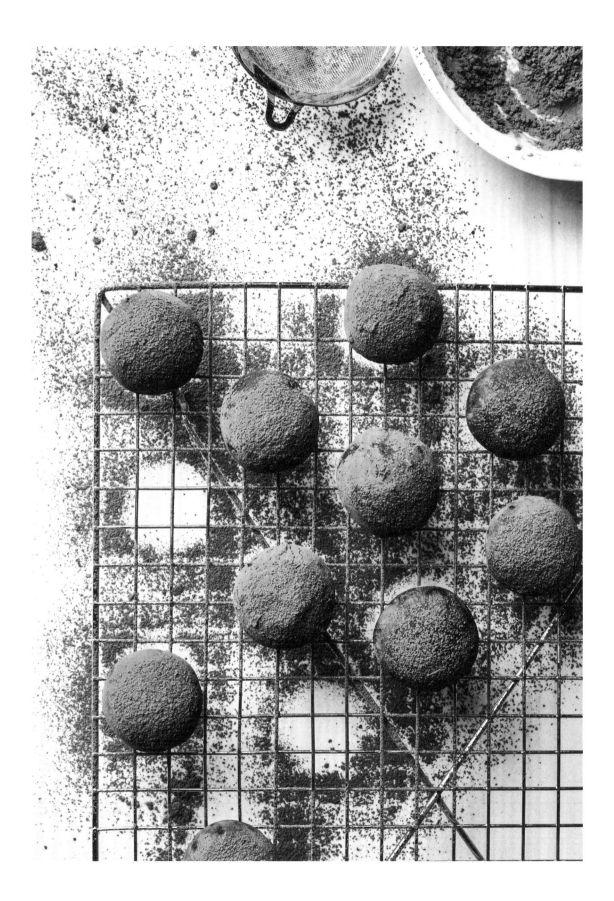

Dairy-Free ◆ Gluten-Free ◆ Grain-Free ◆ Paleo-Friendly Option ◆ Vegetarian ◆ *Makes 8 balls*

Almond Butter Marzipan Balls

Around the holidays, we always visit the Christmas market and pick up marzipan stollen—a sweet German bread with an almond paste filling. Curious how marzipan was made, I began experimenting at home, creating this version that uses honey in place of white sugar. The recipe uses three different forms of almond: almond flour, almond butter, and almond extract to get the signature marzipan flavour. You can serve these marzipan balls to guests at a holiday party or enjoy them all by yourself!

1 cup (250 mL) super-fine blanched almond flour

2 tablespoons (30 mL) natural almond butter or Homemade Almond Butter (page 275)

2 tablespoons (30 mL) raw liquid honey

1½ teaspoons (7 mL) pure almond extract

1 tablespoon (15 mL) raw cacao powder

1. In a medium bowl, combine the almond flour, almond butter, honey, and almond extract. Using your hands, form the mixture into a ball.
2. Transfer to a cutting board and form the ball into a log shape. Slice into 8 portions, then roll each portion into a ball.
3. Arrange a rack on a baking sheet. Transfer the balls to the rack. Using a fine mesh strainer, sift the cocoa powder over the balls, turning them to coat completely. Store in an airtight container in the fridge for up to 1 month.

◆ **Paleo-Friendly:** Skip the pure almond extract.

Sebastian's German Cherry Cake

This recipe is adapted from a traditional German cherry cake called *kirschplotzer*. My husband, Sebastian, grew up in Germany with cherry trees in his backyard, and his family would pick fresh cherries to make this cake. This version is made with canned cherries, so you can make it all year round! The cherries make the cake very moist and juicy, while the rusks lend the cake its bread pudding–like texture. Rusks are hard, dry biscuits that are commonly eaten in Europe. You can find them hidden in the cracker aisle at most grocery stores.

9 ounces (250 g) rusks

2¼ cups (550 mL) unsweetened almond milk

¾ cup (175 mL) ghee or Plain Jane Ghee (page 271), at room temperature

1 cup (250 mL) coconut sugar

5 teaspoons (25 mL) baking powder

1 tablespoon (15 mL) cinnamon

4 pasture-raised or organic eggs

3 cans (14 ounces/400 mL each) sweet cherries, syrup drained

1 teaspoon (5 mL) icing sugar, to serve (optional)

1. Position a rack in the middle of the oven. Preheat the oven to 350°F (180°C). Line the bottom of a 10-inch (3 L) springform pan with parchment paper.

2. In a large bowl, add the rusks and almond milk. Using your hands (and some elbow grease), break up the rusks until they disintegrate into a paste.

3. In a medium bowl, cream together the ghee and coconut sugar. Transfer to the bowl with the rusk mixture. Add the baking powder, cinnamon, and eggs. Stir to combine.

4. Carefully fold in the cherries, ensuring that they are evenly distributed throughout the batter. Pour the batter into the pan, spreading it out evenly with a spatula. Bake until a golden-brown crust forms on top and a toothpick inserted in the centre comes out clean, 1 to 1½ hours.

5. Let sit for 1 hour before removing the cake from the pan. Dust with the icing sugar, if using. Slice and serve. Store the cake covered in the fridge for up to 1 week.

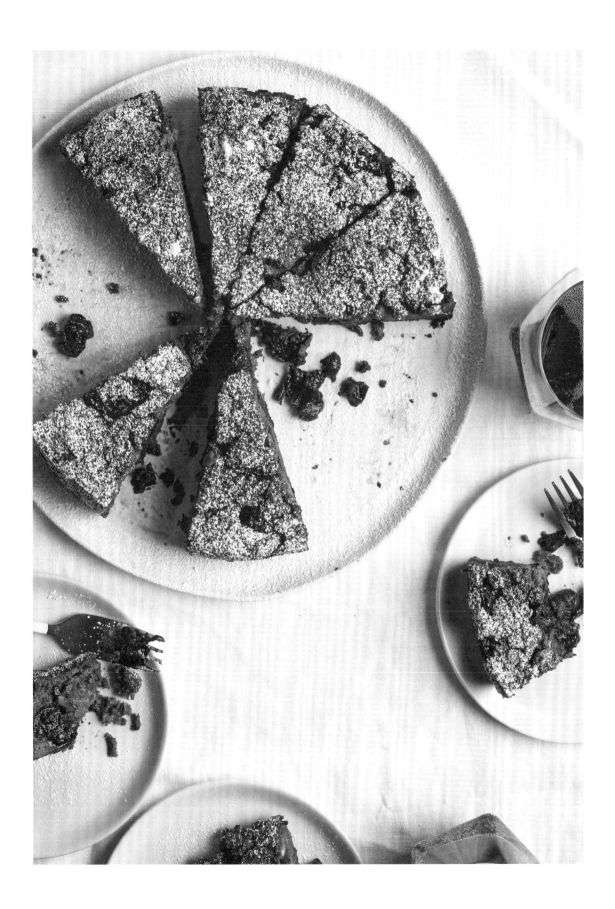

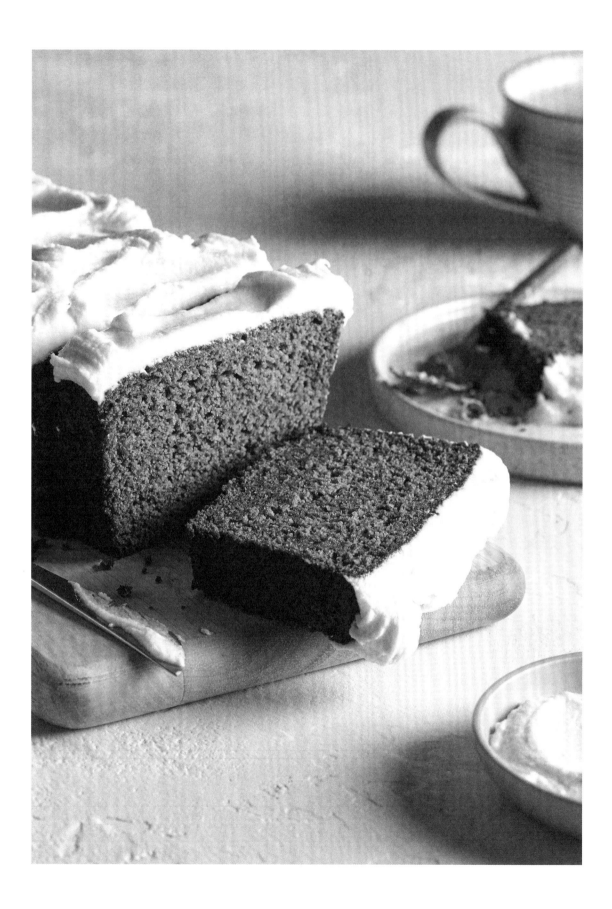

Cardamom Date Cake with Goat Cheese Frosting

This moist date cake is a real crowd-pleaser and is the perfect thing to serve for a fall brunch or an afternoon coffee break. The contrast between the cardamom-spiced cake and the tangy frosting is heavenly! If your dates are older, I recommend soaking them in boiling water for 10 minutes to soften them, so that they are easier to blend.

Cardamom Date Cake

10 soft Medjool dates, pitted

1 cup (250 mL) water

½ cup (125 mL) ghee, Plain Jane Ghee (page 271), or organic unsalted butter, at room temperature

¾ cup (175 mL) coconut sugar

2 pasture-raised or organic eggs

1½ cups (375 mL) sprouted or light spelt flour

1 teaspoon (5 mL) ground cardamom

1 teaspoon (5 mL) cinnamon

1 teaspoon (5 mL) baking soda

1 teaspoon (5 mL) baking powder

Pinch of sea salt

Goat Cheese Frosting

4 ounces (115 g) soft goat cheese

¼ cup (60 mL) ghee, Plain Jane Ghee (page 271), or organic unsalted butter, at room temperature

3 tablespoons (45 mL) raw liquid honey

1. Preheat the oven to 350°F (180°C). Grease a 9- × 5-inch (2 L) loaf pan with ghee.

2. **Make the Cardamom Date Cake** In a high-speed blender or a food processor, combine the dates and water. Blend on high speed into a smooth paste, 15 to 20 seconds.

3. In a large bowl, cream together the ghee and coconut sugar. Add the eggs and the date paste. Whisk to combine.

4. Add the spelt flour, cardamom, cinnamon, baking soda, baking powder, and salt. Fold to combine.

5. Scrape the batter into the loaf pan. Bake until the top is dark golden brown and a toothpick inserted in the centre comes out clean, 45 to 55 minutes. Place the pan on a rack and let cool completely, 1 to 1½ hours.

6. **Make the Goat Cheese Frosting** In a large bowl, add the goat cheese, ghee, and honey. Using electric beaters, beat until stiff peaks form, 4 to 5 minutes.

7. Using a spatula, ice the top of the cake generously with Goat Cheese Frosting and serve. Cover the cake and store in the fridge for up to 1 week. Bring the cake back to room temperature before serving.

Molten Chocolate Lava Cakes

I learned to make lava cakes during a Zen cooking retreat in Germany, and I could not believe how easy and impressive they were. This is a fat-fuelled, gluten-free, dairy-free version that I love. These lava cakes are creamy and rich but not overly sweet. Just be careful not to overcook the cakes, or you won't have any lava in the middle!

7 ounces (200 g) 70% dark chocolate, roughly chopped

1 cup (250 mL) ghee or Plain Jane Ghee (page 271), more for greasing the custard cups, at room temperature

⅓ cup (75 mL) coconut sugar

2½ teaspoons (12 mL) cassava flour

3 pasture-raised or organic eggs

3 pasture-raised or organic egg yolks

1 cup (250 mL) coconut cream, skimmed from 1 can (14 ounces/400 mL) full-fat coconut milk, refrigerated overnight

Coconut Whipped Cream (page 274), to serve (optional)

1. Position a rack in the middle of the oven. Preheat the oven to 350°F (180°C). Grease six 6-ounce (170 g) custard cups with ghee.

2. Using a double boiler or a large heat-proof bowl set over a medium saucepan, bring 2 cups (500 mL) of water to a simmer over medium heat.

3. Add the dark chocolate and ghee to the bowl over the simmering water. Cook, stirring constantly, until completely melted and smooth, 5 to 8 minutes.

4. Add the coconut sugar and flour. Whisk until smooth. One at a time, add the eggs and egg yolks to the bowl, whisking to incorporate before adding the next.

5. Add the coconut cream and stir until smooth. Divide the mixture among the custard cups.

6. Place the cups directly on the rack in the oven. Bake until the sides of the cakes are firm but the centres are still very soft to the touch, 14 to 16 minutes.

7. Gently loosen the cakes around the edges and invert them onto plates. Serve immediately, with Coconut Whipped Cream (if using) on the side.

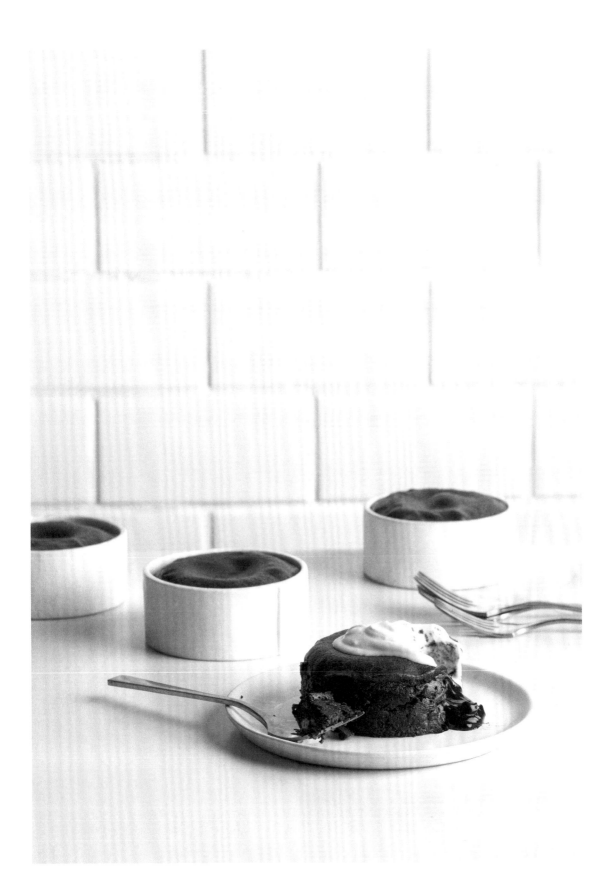

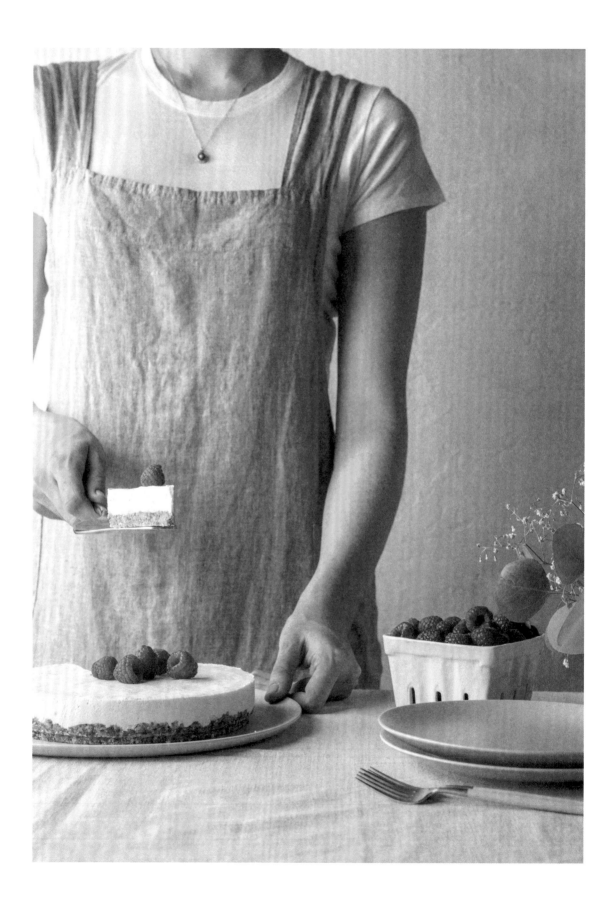

◆ Lemon Ricotta Cheesecake

When I was growing up, my mother would always make cheesecake, which got me totally hooked! To satisfy my cheesecake addiction as an adult, I developed this healthier version that is sweetened with honey and full of good fats from sheep's milk ricotta, coconut cream, and macadamia nuts. It is light, lemony, and fresh—the perfect dessert to please a cheesecake-loving crowd.

Macadamia Nut Crust

8 soft Medjool dates, pitted

1 cup (250 mL) raw macadamia nuts

¼ cup (60 mL) unsweetened shredded coconut

½ teaspoon (2 mL) sea salt

Lemon Ricotta Filling

1½ cups (375 mL) sheep's milk ricotta cheese

1 cup (250 mL) coconut cream, skimmed from 1 can (14 ounces/400 mL) full-fat coconut milk, refrigerated overnight

⅓ cup (75 mL) raw liquid honey

Zest of 1 lemon

⅓ cup (75 mL) fresh lemon juice

1 teaspoon (5 mL) pure vanilla extract

1 pint (2 cups/500 mL) fresh raspberries, to serve

1. Line the bottom of an 8-inch (2 L) springform pan with parchment paper.

2. **Make the Macadamia Nut Crust** In a food processor, add the dates, macadamia nuts, shredded coconut, and salt. Pulse until the mixture sticks together when squeezed in the palm of your hand, 20 to 30 seconds.

3. Using your hands, press the mixture evenly onto the bottom of the prepared pan. Wipe clean the food processor bowl. Place the pan in the freezer while you prepare the Lemon Ricotta Filling.

4. **Make the Lemon Ricotta Filling** In a food processor, combine the ricotta, coconut cream, honey, lemon zest, lemon juice, and vanilla. Blend on high speed until smooth, 20 to 30 seconds.

5. Pour the filling into the crust, spreading it out evenly using a spatula. Cover and place the pan in the freezer for at least 1 hour.

6. Remove the cheesecake from the freezer 30 minutes before serving. Top with fresh raspberries. Slice and serve. Store the cheesecake, covered, in the fridge for up to 5 days or in the freezer for up to 1 month.

Dairy-Free ◆ Gluten-Free ◆ Grain-Free ◆ Nut-Free ◆ Keto-Friendly Option
◆ Paleo-Friendly ◆ Vegetarian ◆ *Makes 16 squares*

Salted Chocolate Halva Fudge with Tahini Drizzle

Packed with good fats, this delicious freezer fudge is a perfect treat for anyone who loves tahini. Inspired by the flavours of Middle Eastern halva, I've used tahini and toasted sesame seeds for a nutty crunch that pairs perfectly with chocolate. A sprinkle of flaky sea salt takes this healthy dessert to the next level. Some brands of tahini are very thick, whereas others are thin. I suggest using thin tahini because you can easily drizzle it on just about anything!

¾ cup (175 mL) ghee or Plain Jane Ghee (page 271)

¾ cup (175 mL) coconut butter or virgin coconut oil

¾ cup (175 mL) tahini, more to serve

¾ cup (175 mL) raw cacao powder

¼ cup (60 mL) pure maple syrup

½ teaspoon (2 mL) sea salt

2 tablespoons (30 mL) sesame seeds

Flaky sea salt, to serve (optional)

1. In a small saucepan over low heat, melt the ghee and coconut butter. Remove from the heat. Add the tahini, cacao powder, maple syrup, and salt. Whisk to combine.

2. Transfer the mixture to a glass 8-inch (2 L) square baking dish. Cover and place in the freezer for at least 2 hours.

3. Remove from the freezer and let sit for 10 minutes at room temperature to soften.

4. Meanwhile, heat a dry, medium skillet over medium heat. Add the sesame seeds in a single layer. Toast, tossing occasionally, until the sesame seeds are fragrant and lightly browned, 4 to 5 minutes.

5. To serve, slice the fudge into 16 squares. Drizzle with tahini. Sprinkle with toasted sesame seeds and flaky sea salt, if using. Enjoy immediately. Store the fudge in an airtight container in the freezer for up to 1 month.

◆ **Keto-Friendly:** Skip the maple syrup or use sugar-free maple syrup from monk fruit sweetener instead.

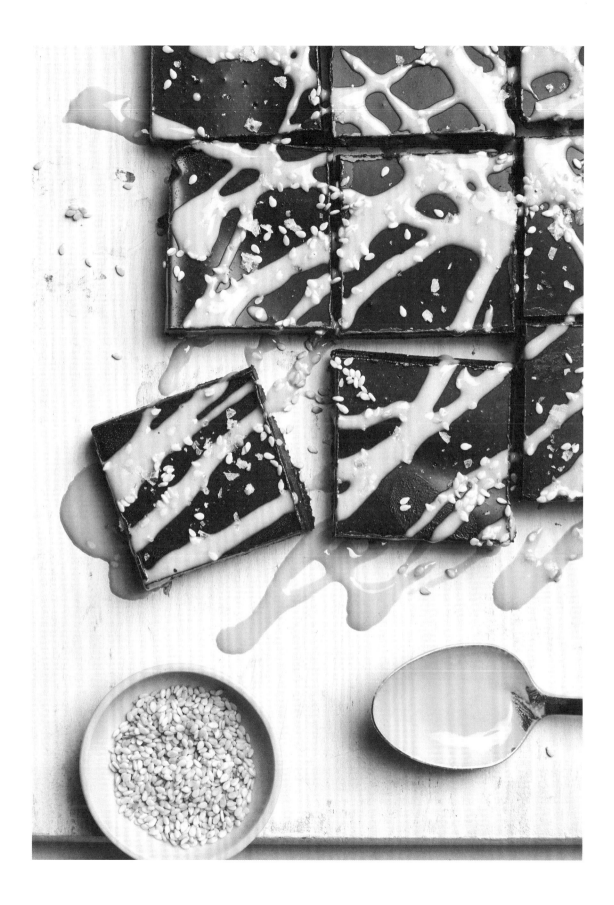

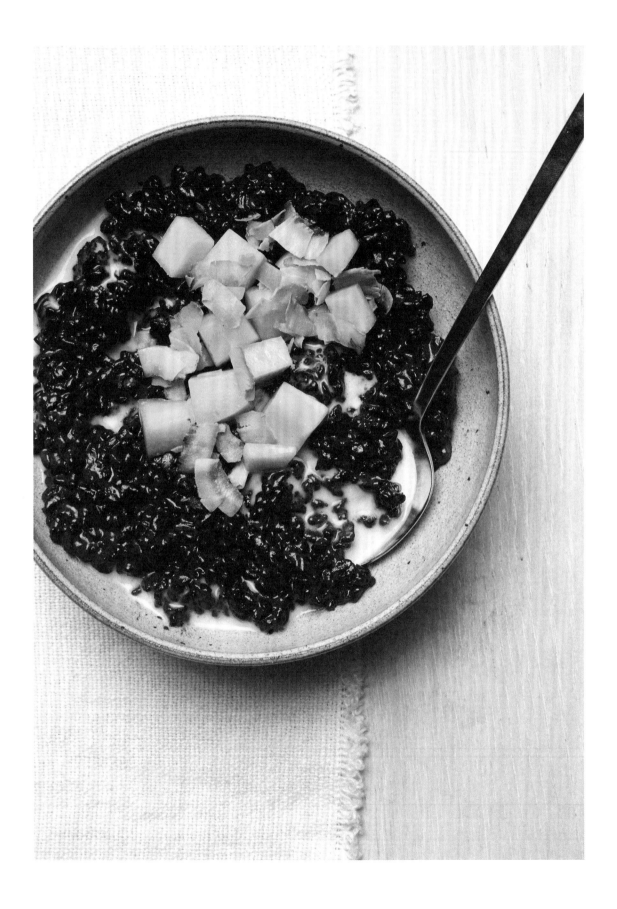

Coconut Black Rice Pudding

This exotic dessert makes me feel like I am somewhere tropical, even if it is the middle of winter in Canada. Coconut is truly the star of the show here, and it's used in the forms of coconut milk, coconut sugar, and toasted coconut flakes. Black forbidden rice (available at specialty stores) adds a lovely earthy flavour and chewy texture. The contrast of the black rice with the white coconut milk and orange-fleshed fruit is beautiful. Any leftover pudding is delicious for breakfast!

1 cup (250 mL) black forbidden rice

¼ teaspoon (1 mL) sea salt

⅓ cup (75 mL) coconut sugar

1 can (14 ounces/400 mL) full-fat coconut milk, divided

½ cup (125 mL) unsweetened coconut flakes

1 cup (250 mL) chopped fresh mango

1. In a medium saucepan, bring 2¼ cups (550 mL) of water to a boil. When the water is boiling, add the black rice and salt. Reduce to a simmer over medium-low heat. Cover and cook, stirring occasionally, until the rice is soft and chewy, 35 to 40 minutes.

2. Add the coconut sugar and 1 cup (250 mL) of the coconut milk to the saucepan. Stir to combine. Cover and simmer, stirring occasionally, until thickened, 15 to 20 minutes. Remove from the heat.

3. Meanwhile, preheat the oven to 325°F (160°C). Line a baking sheet with parchment paper.

4. Spread the coconut flakes in a single layer on the prepared baking sheet. Toast until fragrant and lightly browned, 4 to 6 minutes.

5. To serve, divide the rice pudding among bowls. Top with the mango, toasted coconut, and a splash of the remaining coconut milk. Serve warm. Store leftover rice pudding in an airtight container in the fridge for up to 4 days.

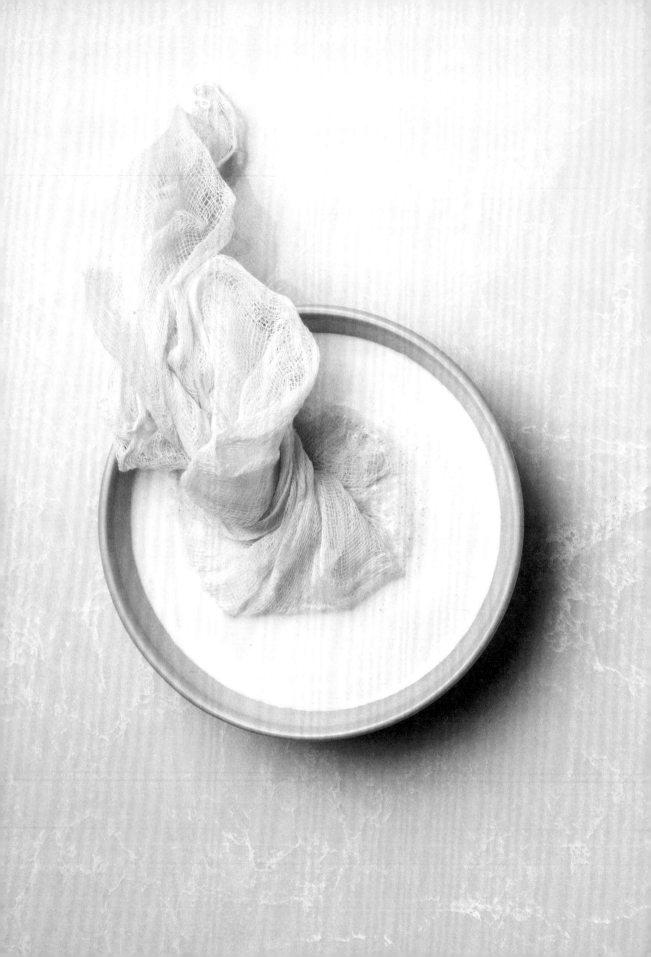

Staples

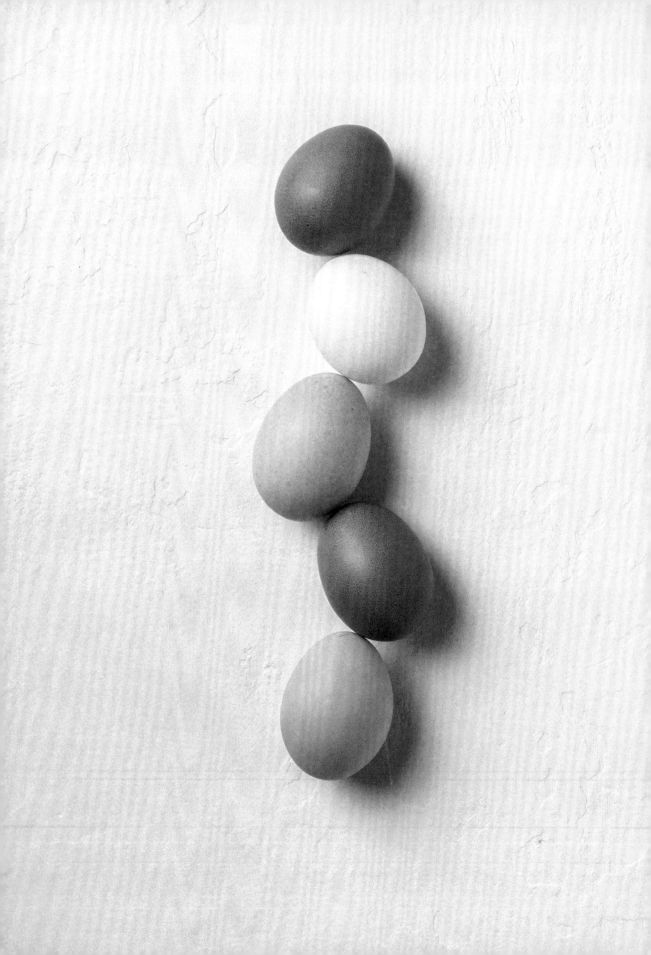

Eggs
Three
Ways

Put an egg on it! Eggs are a great way to amp up the nutrients of any meal. They are full of good fats, vitamins, and choline—a nutrient that is essential for brain function. Look for eggs that are preferably pasture-raised, which means the hens were able to roam freely outdoors and forage on their natural diet. This produces those beautiful orange yolks that are full of omega-3 fatty acids. In a pinch, organic eggs will do the trick. Here are the three methods I use to cook my eggs; use them to top grain bowls, salads, and steaks, or enjoy them all on their own!

Dairy-Free ◆ Gluten-Free ◆ Grain-Free ◆ Keto-Friendly
◆ Nut-Free ◆ Paleo-Friendly ◆ Vegetarian ◆ *Makes 1 egg*

◆ Poached Eggs

Poaching eggs is a great way to get a soft, runny yolk that you can break over the top of your favourite dishes. Poaching also happens to be one of the healthiest ways to cook eggs, because it gently cooks them without the risk of oxidizing the yolk. It is best to use farm-fresh eggs for poaching, as this makes them hold together well. My favourite way to use them is to top the Power Greens Breakfast (page 72). Eating eggs and greens together helps you absorb more nutrients than you would otherwise.

1 pasture-raised or organic egg

1. Fill a medium saucepan half-full with water and bring to a boil over high heat. Reduce to a gentle simmer over medium heat, with only a few small bubbles coming to the surface now and then.

2. Crack the egg into a small bowl.

3. Using a spoon, gently stir the water in the saucepan to create a vortex-like motion. Slide the egg from the bowl into the centre of the vortex. Set a timer for 3 minutes.

4. Using a slotted spoon, remove the egg and test for doneness by gently poking the yolk. It should feel soft and runny on the inside. If you want it cooked more, place it back in the water for another minute. Serve warm.

Jammy Eggs

This is an eight-minute soft-boiled egg that is *jammy* in the centre yet firm around the edges. It is perfect for eating as a snack, sprinkled with flaky sea salt and za'atar, or used to top salads like the Chicken Cobb Salad (page 95) and Wild Salmon Niçoise (page 106). I suggest making several in advance, then peeling and refrigerating them for meals throughout the week. It is best to use grocery store eggs for soft-boiling, as farm-fresh eggs can be harder to peel.

4 to 8 pasture-raised or organic eggs

1. Fill a medium saucepan half-full with water and bring to a boil over high heat.
2. Using a slotted spoon, carefully lower in the desired number of eggs. Boil, uncovered, for exactly 8 minutes. Meanwhile, prepare a bowl of ice water.
3. Using the slotted spoon, remove the eggs from the boiling water and place them immediately in the ice water. Let sit for 5 minutes.
4. Carefully peel off the shells and slice the eggs in halves or quarters. Serve cold or warm.

Ghee-Fried Eggs

If you haven't tried frying your eggs in ghee before, you are in for a treat! The ghee adds an irresistible buttery flavour and makes the eggs nice and crispy around the edges. I like to make these as a simple breakfast alongside sliced avocado and tomato or use them to top Brassica Bibimbap Bowls with Wild Salmon (page 163) and Rainbow Pesto Grain Bowls (page 164).

2 tablespoons (30 mL) ghee or Plain Jane Ghee (page 271)

4 pasture-raised or organic eggs

Sea salt and black pepper, to taste

1. In a large skillet over medium-high heat, melt the ghee.
2. Carefully crack the eggs, one at a time, into the pan (they should sizzle immediately). Cook until the whites are nearly fully set but the yolk is still runny, 2 to 3 minutes.
3. Season with salt and pepper. Tilt the skillet toward you so that the ghee pools at the edge of the pan. Spoon some hot ghee over the egg whites, avoiding the yolks (the whites should bubble up and become fully set). Serve warm.

Dairy-Free ◆ Gluten-Free ◆ Grain-Free ◆ Keto-Friendly
◆ Nut-Free ◆ Paleo-Friendly ◆ *Makes up to 1 pound (450 g)*

Perfect Oven Bacon

This bacon is cooked in the oven, which means less cleanup and perfect bacon every time! No flipping required. Just put it on a baking sheet, pop it in the oven, set the timer, and it is done in no time. This trick will seriously change your life, and you will not go back to using the stovetop method. I buy my bacon at the farmers market and cook it during my weekly meal prep, to add to wraps, salads, and grain bowls during the week.

4 slices to 1 pound (450 g)
organic bacon

1. Preheat the oven to 425°F (220°C).
2. Arrange the bacon in a single layer on an unlined baking sheet. Bake until desired crispiness is reached, 15 to 18 minutes.
3. Using tongs, transfer the bacon to a plate lined with paper towel to absorb the oil. Store the cooked bacon in a resealable container in the fridge for up to 4 days.

Plain Jane Ghee

Ghee is my favourite ingredient to cook with at home! It has a wonderfully buttery flavour, and the high smoke point makes it super versatile. Traditionally used in Indian cooking, ghee is now widely embraced as a healthier butter replacement for baking, adding to lattes, and using as a spread! The trick to making ghee at home is to slowly simmer the butter for a very long time over low heat, without letting it burn. This ensures that all the milk solids properly separate from the fat and helps it develop a nuttier flavour.

1 pound (450 g) unsalted organic butter, cut into 1-inch (2.5 cm) cubes

1. In a medium saucepan over medium-low heat, melt the butter. Simmer, uncovered, stirring occasionally and keeping an eye on the ghee, 35 to 40 minutes. Occasionally, use a spoon to skim off some of the foamy white milk solids that form on the surface of the butter. This prevents the possibility of overflowing the pan.

2. When the liquid has become *completely* clear and golden yellow, and you can see that the milk solids on the bottom of the pan have turned a dark brown, remove from the heat. If the liquid is still cloudy or the milk solids on the bottom of the pan are still white, keep simmering.

3. Meanwhile, line a small fine mesh strainer with 3 layers of cheesecloth. Set the strainer over a tempered glass jar.

4. Carefully pour the ghee through the cheesecloth and strain it into the jar. All the milk solids should get trapped in the cheesecloth, and the liquid in the jar should be completely clear. If the strained liquid still has milk solids in it, strain it again.

5. Let the ghee solidify at room temperature before sealing the jar. Store at room temperature for up to 3 months or in the fridge for up to 1 year. To prolong the shelf life, always use a clean utensil to dip into the jar and close the lid after each use.

◆ Bone Broth

Bone broth is a nourishing broth made by simmering high-quality bones with aromatics and vegetables for 24 to 48 hours. This recipe can be made with organic chicken bones or grass-fed beef bones; both types of bones can be bought at any reputable butcher shop. Bone broth is full of collagen protein, which is beneficial for your gut, skin, hair, and nails and helps replenish our body's declining collagen as we age. The broth can be used in place of store-bought broth to amp up the flavour and nutritional value of dishes.

2 pounds (900 g) organic chicken bones or grass-fed beef bones

2 tablespoons (30 mL) apple cider vinegar

1 medium yellow onion, peeled and quartered

1 head of garlic, peeled

3 carrots, peeled and roughly chopped

2 stalks of celery, roughly chopped

3 bay leaves

1 teaspoon (5 mL) sea salt

½ teaspoon (2 mL) black peppercorns

1. Fill a stock pot with 4 quarts (4 L) of water. Add the chicken or beef bones and apple cider vinegar. Cover and bring to a boil over high heat. Reduce the heat to medium-low and simmer, covered, for 30 minutes. Using a large spoon or a fine mesh strainer, occasionally skim off and discard the grey foam that forms on the surface of the liquid.

2. Add the onion, garlic, carrots, celery, bay leaves, salt, and peppercorns. Cover and simmer over medium-low heat for 24 hours for chicken broth or 48 hours for beef broth.

3. Using a fine mesh strainer, strain the broth into a large heat-safe pitcher (I use the jar of my blender for this purpose). Discard the solids.

4. Pour the broth into tempered glass jars, leaving 1 inch (2.5 cm) of headspace. Let cool completely before sealing the jars. Store in the fridge for up to 7 days or in the freezer for up to 3 months.

◆ **Tip:** To make this broth in an Instant Pot, use the sauté function to simmer the bones, water, and apple cider vinegar for 30 minutes, skimming off the grey foam that forms on the surface. Add the onion, garlic, carrots, celery, bay leaves, salt, and peppercorns. Set the Instant Pot to high pressure. Set the timer for 2 hours for chicken bones and 4 hours for beef bones. Use a quick pressure release, then strain and transfer to jars. Store as described in the recipe.

Dairy-Free ◆ Gluten-Free ◆ Grain-Free ◆ Keto-Friendly ◆ Paleo-Friendly ◆ Vegan ◆ *Makes 4 cups (1 L)*

Nut Milk

Nut milk is an excellent alternative to dairy milk that can be used in cooking, baking, smoothies, and lattes. Making nut milk at home is a great way to save money, and the result is a much tastier, healthier product than you can find in stores. You can use almonds or macadamia nuts in this recipe—the latter are creamier, more delicious, and more precious. I like to save leftover almond pulp to make Seedy Almond Pulp Crackers (page 192) so that nothing goes to waste.

1¼ cups (300 mL) raw whole almonds or macadamia nuts

4 cups (1 L) filtered water

Pinch of sea salt

1. In a medium bowl, cover the nuts with room-temperature water and soak for at least 1 hour. Drain and rinse.
2. In a high-speed blender, combine the soaked nuts, filtered water, and salt. Blend on high speed until smooth, 1 to 2 minutes.
3. Using a nut milk bag, strain the mixture over a large bowl. Squeeze the bag to extract as much liquid as possible.
4. Pour the nut milk into a 1-quart (1 L) mason jar. Cover and store in the fridge for up to 5 days. Reserve the almond pulp to make Seedy Almond Pulp Crackers (page 192).

◆ **Tip:** To use macadamia pulp to make Seedy Macadamia Pulp Crackers, you will need to collect pulp over 2 or 3 batches of macadamia milk. Macadamia nuts are less fibrous than almonds and therefore produce less pulp.

Dairy-Free ◆ Gluten-Free ◆ Grain-Free ◆ Nut-Free ◆ Keto-Friendly Option
◆ Paleo-Friendly Option ◆ Vegan ◆ *Makes 1 cup (250 mL)*

Coconut Whipped Cream

This is a fat-fuelled whipped cream made from coconut milk that I serve with Sourdough French Toast with Bacon (page 51), Grain-Free Peach Almond Crumble (page 245), Molten Chocolate Lava Cakes (page 256), or anytime I feel a bit indulgent. It is so simple to make and happens to be dairy-free, making it a great option to serve to guests who can't have dairy.

1 cup (250 mL) coconut cream, skimmed from 1 can (14 ounces/400 mL) full-fat coconut milk, refrigerated overnight

1 tablespoon (15 mL) pure maple syrup

¼ teaspoon (1 mL) pure vanilla extract or a pinch of pure vanilla powder

1. Place a medium metal bowl and metal beaters in the freezer for 20 minutes to chill.

2. In the chilled bowl, add the coconut cream. Using electric beaters, beat continuously on high speed until stiff peaks form, 4 to 5 minutes.

3. Add the maple syrup and vanilla. Gently stir to combine. Refrigerate until ready to serve.

◆ **Keto-Friendly:** Skip the maple syrup or use sugar-free maple syrup from monk fruit sweetener instead. Use pure vanilla powder instead of pure vanilla extract.
Paleo-Friendly: Use pure vanilla powder instead of pure vanilla extract.

274 EAT GOOD FAT

Dairy-Free ◆ Gluten-Free ◆ Grain-Free ◆ Keto-Friendly
◆ Paleo-Friendly ◆ Vegan ◆ *Makes 1¼ cups (300 mL)*

◆ Homemade Almond Butter

This is a simple, foolproof almond butter recipe that works every time. Almond butter is a staple in many of the recipes in this book because of its healthy fats and protein. It adds a nutty flavour, creamy texture, and dose of healthy fats to meals. Drizzle it on oatmeal, smoothies, roasted vegetables, noodle dishes, and desserts. If you are feeling indulgent, I suggest adding a pinch of pure vanilla powder. You will not be able to resist eating it straight out of the jar.

2½ cups (625 mL) raw whole almonds

¼ teaspoon (1 mL) sea salt

Pinch of pure vanilla powder (optional)

1. Preheat the oven to 350°F (180°C).
2. Arrange the almonds in a single layer on an unlined baking sheet. Roast until fragrant, 8 to 10 minutes. Let cool for 10 minutes.
3. Transfer the almonds to a food processor. Process on medium speed continuously, until smooth and creamy (this takes time, so be patient). If your food processor starts to overheat, take a break for a minute or two. This process can take anywhere from 10 to 20 minutes, depending on the power of your food processor and how many breaks you need to take.
4. Add the salt and vanilla powder (if using) and pulse to combine. Transfer to an airtight container and store in the fridge for up to 1 month.

◆ Fresh Pesto

This is my favourite pesto recipe—bursting with fresh, vibrant flavour and healthy fats from olive oil, nuts, and raw sheep's milk cheese. Use it on sandwiches, burgers, grain bowls, pizzas, pasta, and vegetables—and anywhere else you can think of! I love the classic pine nut version, but you can substitute whichever nuts you have on hand.

½ cup (125 mL) raw pine nuts

⅔ cup (150 mL) grated pecorino cheese

1 clove garlic, finely grated

⅔ cup (150 mL) extra-virgin olive oil

1 teaspoon (5 mL) sea salt

4 cups (1 L) loosely packed fresh basil leaves, roughly chopped

1. Heat a dry, medium skillet over medium-low heat. Add the pine nuts in a single layer. Toast, tossing frequently, until fragrant and lightly browned, 3 to 5 minutes.

2. In a food processor, combine the toasted pine nuts, pecorino, garlic, olive oil, and salt. Blend on medium speed until the nuts are finely ground, about 30 seconds. Add the basil and process for 30 seconds, until the pesto is smooth. Store in an airtight container in the fridge for up to 3 weeks.

Dairy-Free ◆ Gluten-Free ◆ Grain-Free ◆ Nut-Free ◆ Keto-Friendly
◆ Paleo-Friendly ◆ Vegetarian ◆ *Makes 1 cup (250 mL)*

◆ Lemon Aioli

Aioli is a garlic olive oil mayonnaise that is popular in France and Spain. You need to use room-temperature eggs so that the mayonnaise will emulsify correctly. To get them to room temperature quickly, I simply place the eggs in a bowl of warm water for 5 to 7 minutes. I love using this zesty condiment to add creaminess to my Salmon Avocado Club Wraps (page 155), Easy Salmon Salad (page 109), and Grain-Free Everything Bagels with Smoked Trout Spread (page 67). It is also heavenly on steamed vegetables, Jammy Eggs (page 269), and poached fish! This recipe has raw egg in it, so it isn't recommended for small children, pregnant women, or the elderly.

2 organic, pasture-raised eggs, at room temperature

⅔ cup (150 mL) + 1 tablespoon (15 mL) avocado oil, divided

⅓ cup (75 mL) extra-virgin olive oil

2 teaspoons (10 mL) Dijon mustard

1 clove garlic

¼ teaspoon (1 mL) sea salt

Zest of 1 lemon

3 tablespoons (45 mL) fresh lemon juice

1. Separate the yolk from one of the eggs. The yolk will help the aioli emulsify and become creamier. Save the egg white for another use.

2. In a glass liquid measuring cup or other small pitcher, combine ⅔ cup (150 mL) of the avocado oil with the olive oil.

3. In a food processor, combine the remaining whole egg, egg yolk, mustard, garlic, salt, and the remaining 1 tablespoon (15 mL) avocado oil. On low speed over 1 to 2 minutes, very slowly and in a thin, steady, continuous stream, pour in the oil mixture.

4. The aioli should thicken and cling to the sides of the food processor when emulsified.

5. Add the lemon zest and lemon juice. Blend for 10 more seconds. Store in an airtight container in the fridge for up to 3 weeks.

✦ Acknowledgements

It takes a village to write a book, and this book would not have been possible if it were not for the many people who put in countless hours to help see this project through to completion. I am beyond grateful for each and every one of you who shared this journey with me.

To my hubs, Sebastian. Thank you from the bottom of my heart for holding down the fort while I wrote this book. For believing in me, doing all the dishes, shipping out our orders, doing grocery store runs, responding to customer emails, keeping our production records up to date, eating every recipe I made (usually many days in a row), brainstorming recipe ideas into the wee hours of the morning, copy editing, and so, so much more. I couldn't have done this without your love and support. You are truly my hero, and I am so lucky to have you.

To my mum, thank you for teaching me from a young age that you can do anything you set your mind to. Getting here hasn't been easy, but you've been right there with me all along the way, encouraging me, supporting me, and lifting me up whenever things got hard. It is because of your strength and support that I can overcome any challenges that come my way.

To my dad, I hope I've made you very proud. To Rachel, Savannah, Max, Kasia, Matt, Adelaide, and Dinah, thank you for being with me on every step of this adventure. I am so grateful to have all of you on my team.

To Pat and Forbes, thank you for hosting me while I honed my knife skills at Le Cordon Bleu. To Bill and Barb, thank you for your legal expertise and for being my most loyal customers.

To Thea Baumann, my chief recipe tester who spent most of her pregnancy with twins recreating the recipes in this book, and somehow managed to finish testing them after her daughters were born. Thank you for your hard work, dedication, and very detailed notes.

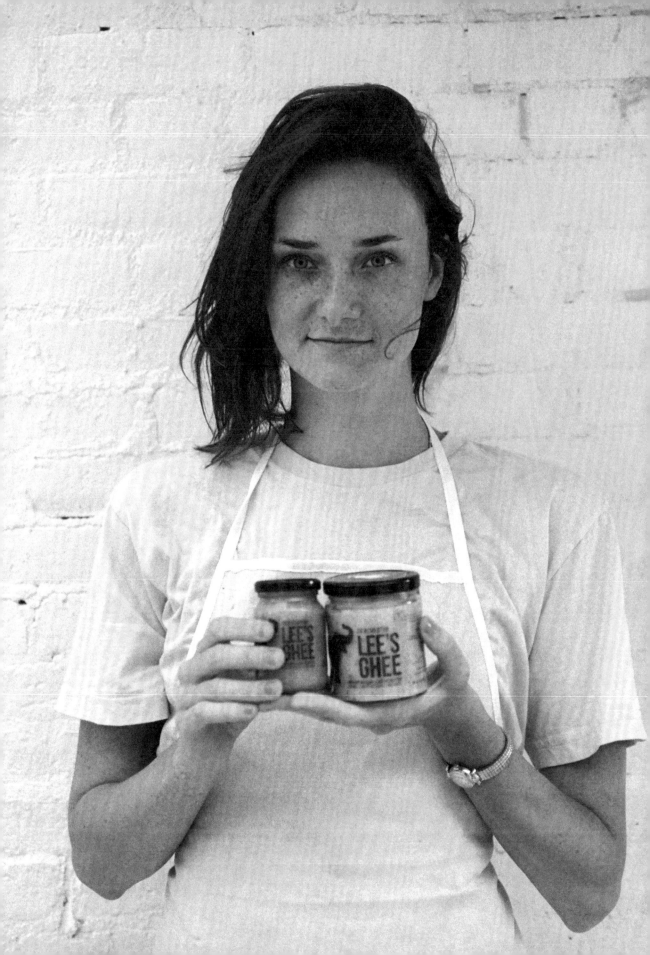

To Kaitlin, Dave, Jessica, Noah, Sarah, Holly, Paul, Eladia, Ben, Genevieve, Deb, Catherine, Ashleigh, Phillis, Rosanne, Jaclyn, Michael, Jorge, Nanci, Karen, Savannah, and Rachel, thank you for recreating my recipes and sharing your honest feedback with me. You are all shining stars.

To my creative team, Lauren Miller, Dara Sutin, and Rayna Marlee, who helped bring my vision to life. You guys are so talented, and it was an honour to work with you. Thank you for your dedication to making this book even more beautiful than I ever could have imagined.

To Julia Gibson, thank you for your nutrition wisdom and cooking skills, managing our social media accounts, and helping out whenever I needed an extra hand—literally!

Thank you to the team at Evergreen Brick Works, who allowed me time away from the farmers market to write this book. And thank you to the many farmers who worked hard to grow the food used to develop the recipes in this book—I can assure you that nothing went to waste.

To Andrea Magyar, my editor, thank you for believing in me and sharing my vision. You have been so helpful and supportive throughout this process. Thank you to the rest of the Penguin Random House Canada team for everything you have done to make this book come to life.

To Rick Broadhead, my literary agent, thank you for not thinking I was crazy for wanting to write a book about fat and for giving me the confidence to put my ideas into writing. Thank you also to Joe Mimran, for introducing us.

Last but not least, thank you to all of my customers. Every time someone sends me a kind email, writes a glowing review, or posts a recipe made with my ghee, I am reminded of the fantastic community that supports what I am doing and allows me to do what I love. For that, I am eternally grateful. Thank you for inspiring me to write this book—this book is for you.

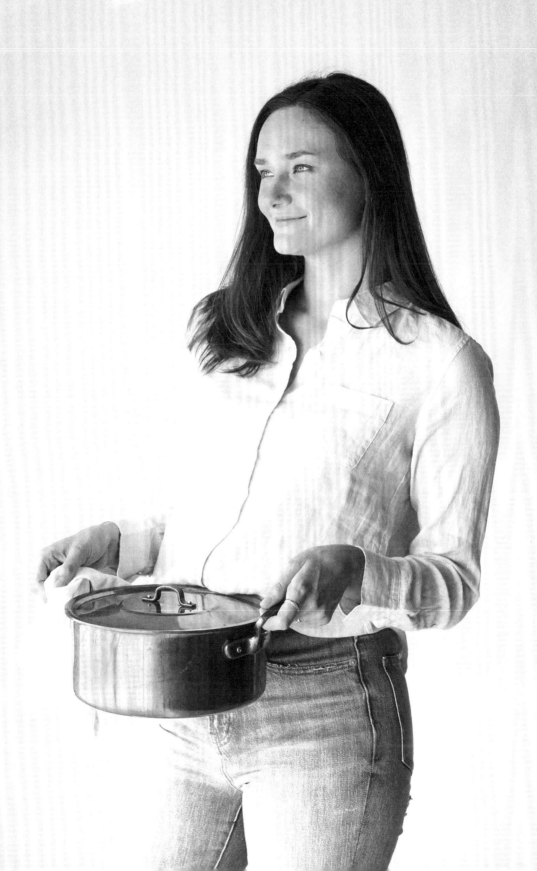

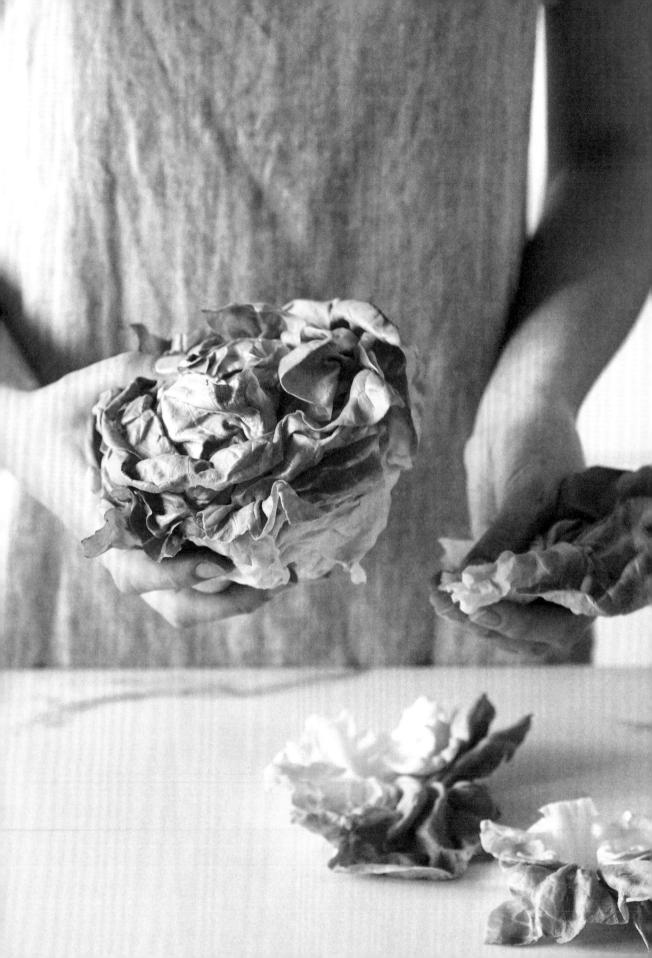

✦ Index